The Easy Veg Keto 5-Ingredient Diet Cookbook

170+ High-Fat, Low-Carb, Dairy-free, Egg-free Recipes for Busy People on the Plant based Keto Diet with 4 weeks meal plan

John Ami

ISBN: 9798864090381

DEDICATION

Dedicated to as many who Looking for a cookbook that combines the benefits of a vegan and ketogenic diet with simple, easy-to-follow recipes

TABLE OF CONTENTS

INTRODUCTION

The high-fat, low-carb, dairy-free, egg-free vegan keto diet is a powerful nutritional approach that combines the principles of veganism and ketogenic eating. By focusing on plant-based, whole food sources rich in healthy fats and low in carbohydrates, this diet offers a myriad of benefits. Firstly, it promotes weight loss and improved metabolic health. By reducing carbohydrate intake, the body shifts into a state of ketosis, where it burns fat for fuel, leading to more effective fat loss. Moreover, this diet supports stable blood sugar levels and reduced inflammation, making it an excellent choice for people with diabetes or those seeking to manage insulin resistance. It's also heart-healthy, as it emphasizes healthy fats like avocados, nuts, and seeds, which can lead to improved cholesterol levels. Additionally, the exclusion of dairy and eggs makes it suitable for those with allergies or dietary restrictions.

Furthermore, this diet encourages a diverse and nutrient-dense plant-based intake, providing ample fiber, antioxidants, and essential nutrients. It's a sustainable and environmentally-friendly choice, aligning with ethical and ecological values. Overall, the high-fat, low-carb, dairy-free, egg-free vegan keto diet is a versatile and effective approach to achieving optimal health and wellness.

Benefits of a 5-Ingredient Approach

A 5-ingredient approach in a ketogenic (keto) vegan diet can offer several benefits, making it easier to maintain the diet while still meeting your nutritional needs. The key advantages include simplicity, adherence, and the promotion of whole, nutrient-dense foods. Here are some benefits of following a 5-ingredient keto vegan diet:

1. Simplicity: A 5-ingredient approach simplifies meal planning and preparation. With fewer ingredients, you spend less time in the kitchen and reduce the likelihood of making errors that could affect your ketosis.

2. Compliance: Keeping your meals limited to just five ingredients can make it easier to stay within the macronutrient ratios required for a ketogenic diet. It helps you avoid hidden carbs and sugars that might be present in more complex recipes.

3. Nutrient Density: Focusing on whole, plant-based ingredients ensures that your diet is rich in vitamins, minerals, and antioxidants. Nuts, seeds, leafy greens, and other plant foods provide essential nutrients that support overall health.

4. Satiety: Many plant-based keto foods, such as avocados, nuts, and seeds, are naturally high in healthy fats and fiber. This combination can help keep you feeling full and satisfied, reducing the temptation to snack on non-keto foods.

5. Digestive Health: A simple, whole-food-based diet can be gentler on the digestive system. Some people experience digestive issues when they consume a lot of complex ingredients or artificial additives, which are often found in processed vegan products.

6. Sustainability: A vegan diet is generally more sustainable and eco-friendly than diets based on animal products. Reducing the number of ingredients in your meals

can further reduce your environmental impact by cutting down on food packaging and processing.

7. Cost-Efficiency: A minimalist approach to ingredients can save you money. Whole foods are often more affordable than specialty vegan products or processed foods.

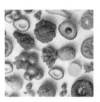

Pantry Staples for a Keto Vegan Diet

Stocking your pantry with the right staples is crucial for maintaining a keto vegan diet. Below are some important pantry items to have on hand:

1. **Nuts and Seeds:** Almonds, walnuts, pecans, macadamia nuts Chia seeds, flax seeds, hemp seeds, sunflower seeds

2. **Nut and Seed Butters:** Almond butter, peanut butter, sunflower seed butter Coconut Products: Coconut oil, coconut milk (unsweetened), shredded coconut

3. Low-Carb Flours: Almond flour, coconut flour, flaxseed meal

4. **Non-Dairy Milks:** Almond milk, coconut milk (unsweetened), hemp milk

5. **Plant-Based Protein Sources:** Tofu, tempeh, edamame, textured vegetable protein (TVP)

6. **Low-Carb Sweeteners:** Stevia, erythritol, monk fruit sweetener

7. **Non-Starchy Vegetables:** Leafy greens (spinach, kale, arugula), broccoli, cauliflower, zucchini, Brussels sprouts

8. **Condiments and Sauces:** Olive oil, avocado oil, vinegar (e.g., apple cider, balsamic) Tamari (gluten-free soy sauce), coconut aminos Mustard, hot sauce, sugar-free ketchup

9. **Herbs, Spices, and Seasonings:** Garlic powder, onion powder, cumin, paprika, turmeric, curry powder
Salt, pepper, basil, oregano, thyme, rosemary

10. Baking Essentials: Baking powder, baking soda, xanthan gum (for gluten-free baking)
Unsweetened cocoa powder (for chocolate recipes)

11. Flavor Enhancers: Nutritional yeast (for a cheesy flavor), miso paste, tahini

12. Canned Goods: Coconut cream, diced tomatoes (no added sugar), tomato paste Artichoke hearts, hearts of palm, olives

13. Non-Dairy Yogurt: Unsweetened coconut or almond milk yogurt

14. Snacks: Seaweed snacks, unsweetened coconut chips, low-carb nuts/seeds

15. Low-Carb Pasta Alternatives: Shirataki noodles, zucchini noodles (zoodles)

16. Sustainable Protein Sources: Legumes (in moderation): Lentils, chickpeas, black soybeans (lower in carbs)

17. Supplements (Optional): B12, Omega-3 (from algae oil), vitamin D (if not getting enough sunlight exposure)

Remember to always check labels for hidden sugars or non-vegan additives. Furthermore, consider your individual dietary needs and preferences. This list provides a good starting point, but feel free to customize it based on what works best for you.

Essential Kitchen Tools

Having the right kitchen tools can make preparing keto vegan meals much easier and more enjoyable. Here's a list of essential kitchen tools for a keto vegan diet:

1. High-Speed Blender: Useful for making smoothies, sauces, soups, and nut-based creams. Look for a durable blender that can handle tough ingredients like nuts and seeds.
2. Food Processor: Great for chopping, shredding, and making nut-based sauces or spreads. It's also useful for making cauliflower rice or zucchini noodles.
3. Spiralizer: Essential for turning vegetables like zucchini or sweet potatoes into noodles, a low-carb alternative to pasta.
4. Non-Stick Frying Pan or Skillet: Choose a high-quality, non-toxic, non-stick pan for cooking vegetables, tofu, and plant-based proteins.
5. Cast Iron Skillet: Ideal for searing, frying, and baking. It provides even heat distribution and can add a nice sear to tofu or vegetable steaks.
6. Chef's Knife and Cutting Board: A sharp knife and a sturdy cutting board are essential for chopping vegetables, fruits, and other ingredients.
7. Baking Sheet or Tray: Useful for roasting vegetables, making keto-friendly snacks, or baking.
8. Pots and Pans: Invest in a set of good-quality pots and pans for boiling, steaming, and cooking soups and stews.
9. Measuring Cups and Spoons: Accurate measurements are crucial for keto recipes, especially when dealing with precise ratios of fats, proteins, and carbohydrates.
10. Mason Jars and Storage Containers: Useful for storing prepped ingredients, sauces, and leftovers.
11. Vegetable Peeler: Handy for peeling and preparing vegetables like zucchini or carrots.
12. Silicone Baking Mats or Parchment Paper: These prevent sticking when baking and roasting without adding extra oil.
13. Tongs and Spatula: Essential for flipping and turning food in a hot pan or on a grill.
14. Micro plane Grater/Zester: Useful for grating citrus zest, garlic, ginger, and hard cheeses.
15. Strainer or Colander: Necessary for draining cooked vegetables or pasta alternatives like shirataki noodles.
16 Can Opener: For opening cans of coconut milk, diced tomatoes, or other canned ingredients.
17. Salad Spinner: Helps clean and dry leafy greens and herbs efficiently.
18. Digital Food Scale: Useful for accurate portion control and tracking macros.
19. Oven Mitts or Heat-Resistant Gloves: Necessary for handling hot pots, pans, and baking dishes.

20. Food Storage Bags and Wraps: Essential for keeping food fresh in the fridge or freezer.

Remember, investing in quality kitchen tools can save you time and effort in the long run, making your keto vegan cooking experience more enjoyable and efficient.

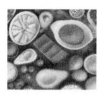

Budget-Friendly Shopping for 5-Ingredient Recipes

Shopping for budget-friendly 5-ingredient recipes requires careful planning and a focus on cost-effective ingredients. Below are some tips for budget-conscious shopping for your keto vegan diet:

1. Plan Your Meals: Before you go shopping, plan your meals for the week. This will help you create a specific shopping list and avoid buying unnecessary items.

2. Stick to Simple Ingredients: Choose recipes that rely on basic, affordable staples like beans, lentils, tofu, leafy greens, and affordable vegetables like cabbage, carrots, and zucchini.

3. Buy in Bulk: Consider buying non-perishable items like nuts, seeds, grains, and dried legumes in bulk. Buying in bulk is generally a more cost-effective approach than purchasing smaller quantities.

4. Choose Frozen or Canned Produce: Frozen fruits and vegetables can be just as nutritious as fresh ones and are usually more affordable. Canned vegetables like tomatoes and beans are also budget-friendly and have a long shelf life.

5. Compare Prices: Pay attention to unit prices (price per ounce or gram) when comparing different brands or package sizes. Sometimes buying a larger quantity is more economical.

6. Shop seasonally and locally: Seasonal produce is often more affordable and tastes better. Additionally, consider shopping at local markets or stores that offer lower prices on fresh produce.

7. Use Store Brands and Generic Labels: Store brands or generic labels are usually cheaper than name-brand products and are often of similar quality.

8. Limit Pre-Packaged and Processed Foods: Pre-packaged and processed foods tend to be more expensive. Always choose whole, unprocessed ingredients whenever available.

9. Utilize Sales and Discounts: Keep an eye on sales, discounts, and promotions. Consider using loyalty cards or shopping during sales events to save money.

10. Buy in Bulk and Freeze: If you find a good deal on perishable items like tofu or vegetables, consider buying in bulk and freezing what you won't use immediately.

11. Repurpose Leftovers: Plan meals that allow you to use ingredients in different ways. For example, use leftover cooked vegetables in a salad or stir-fry the next day.

12. Minimize Waste: Be mindful of food expiration dates and use perishable items before they go bad. Use all parts of a vegetable or fruit, including stems and peels, when possible.

13. Limit Specialty Ingredients: While some specialty ingredients can be beneficial, they can also be expensive. Save them for special occasions and focus on budget-friendly basics for everyday meals.

14. Cook in Batches: Prepare larger quantities of meals and freeze portions for later. This can help reduce food costs in the long run.

15. Consider DIY Staples: Making your own staples like nut butter, vegetable broth, or salad dressings can be more cost-effective than buying them pre-made.

By following these tips and being mindful of your budget, you can create delicious and nutritious 5-ingredient keto vegan meals without breaking the bank.

Maximizing Flavor with Minimal Ingredients

Maximizing flavor with minimal ingredients is a skill that can elevate your cooking, especially in a 5-ingredient keto vegan diet. Here are some techniques to make the most of each ingredient:

1. Use Fresh, High-Quality Ingredients: Fresh produce and high-quality spices and herbs often have more intense flavors. Invest in fresh ingredients whenever possible.

2. Highlight One Star Ingredient: Choose one ingredient to be the star of the dish. This could be a vibrant herb, a bold spice, or a flavorful vegetable. Let it shine in the dish.

3. Experiment with Seasonings and Spices: Even with a limited ingredient list, you can create complex flavors by using a variety of herbs and spices. For example, garlic, ginger, cumin, paprika, and fresh herbs like basil or cilantro can add depth to your dishes.

4. Layer Flavors: Create depth by adding flavors at different stages of cooking. For example, start with aromatics like garlic and onions, then add herbs and spices later in the cooking process.

5. Balance Sweet, Salty, Sour, and Bitter: Aim for a balanced combination of these flavor profiles. For example, a squeeze of lemon or a splash of vinegar can add a touch of acidity, while a pinch of salt can enhance other flavors.

6. Utilize Umami-Rich Ingredients: Ingredients like soy sauce, nutritional yeast, miso paste, and mushrooms add a savory, umami flavor that can enhance the overall taste of your dishes.

7. Incorporate Citrus Zest and Juice: Citrus zest and juice can brighten up the flavors of a dish. The zest contains essential oils that are rich in flavor, while the juice provides a tangy element.

8. Roast and Caramelize Vegetables: Roasting or caramelizing vegetables brings out their natural sweetness and intensifies their flavor. It's a simple technique that can add depth to your dishes.

9. Use Aromatics Wisely: Garlic, ginger, and onions are potent flavor enhancers. Use them judiciously to impart a strong base of flavor to your dishes.

10. Experiment with Different Cooking Techniques: Grilling, roasting, sautéing, and steaming can all bring out unique flavors in your ingredients. Each method can add a different dimension to your dishes.

11. Add Texture Contrast: Combining ingredients with different textures can create a more interesting eating experience. For example, pairing creamy avocado with crunchy nuts or seeds can add depth to a salad.

12. Balance Heat and Spice: If you enjoy spicy food, consider using chili peppers, hot sauce, or dried chili flakes. Use them sparingly to add a kick without overwhelming the other flavors.

13. Finish with Fresh Herbs and Citrus: Adding fresh herbs like parsley, cilantro, or basil at the end of cooking can brighten up the dish. Squeezing a bit of lemon or lime juice can also provide a fresh, zesty finish.

Remember, practice and experimentation are key to becoming proficient at maximizing flavor with minimal ingredients. Start with small adjustments and taste as you go to find the perfect balance for your palate.

Portion Control and Nutritional Balance

Portion control and achieving nutritional balance are crucial aspects of maintaining a healthy keto vegan diet. Here are some tips to help you manage portion sizes and ensure you're getting a well-rounded intake of nutrients:

1. Use Smaller Plates and Bowls: Using smaller dishes can trick your brain into thinking you're eating a larger portion, helping you control your portion sizes.

2. Cultivate Mindful Eating Habits: Listen to your body's natural cues for hunger and satiet. Eat slowly and savor each bite. This can help prevent overeating.

3. Read Labels and Serving Sizes: Pay attention to portion sizes listed on food labels. This can give you a better understanding of how much you're consuming.

4. Divide Your Plate: Aim to fill half of your plate with non-starchy vegetables, one-quarter with protein-rich foods, and one-quarter with healthy fats. This helps ensure a balanced intake of nutrients.

5. Track Your Macros: Make use of food tracking app or journal to keep track of your macronutrient intake. This can help you stay within the desired range for a keto diet.

6. Be Mindful of Snacking: While snacking can be a part of a keto diet, be mindful of portion sizes. Pre-portion snacks to avoid mindless eating.

7. Listen to Your Body: Always pay good attention to how your body feels after eating. If you're still hungry, have a small second serving or a healthy snack. If you're full, stop eating.

8. Include a Variety of Foods: Eating a wide range of fruits, vegetables, nuts, seeds, and plant-based proteins ensures you get a diverse array of nutrients.

9. Prioritize Fiber: Fiber-rich foods like vegetables, fruits, and whole grains can help you feel full and satisfied, making it easier to control portion sizes.

10. Limit Processed Foods: Processed foods can be easy to overeat due to their high palatability. Try as much as possible to limit your intake of processed meals and snacks.

11. Practice Intuitive Eating: Focus on eating when you're hungry and stopping when you're satisfied. Practice mindful eating by avoiding consumption driven by boredom, stress, or emotional cues.

12. Maintain Proper Hydration: Ensure you're adequately hydrated; sometimes your body might signal thirst as hunger. Make sure you're adequately hydrated to avoid overeating.

13. Plan Your Meals: Having a meal plan can help you portion out your ingredients and avoid overindulging.

14. Adjust Portions Based on Activity Level: If you're highly active, you may need larger portions to meet your energy needs. Be mindful of your activity level and adjust portion sizes accordingly.

Finding the right portion sizes for your body may take some trial and error. Pay good attention to how different portion sizes make you feel and try to make adjustment as needed. It's important to find a balance that supports your energy needs and overall well-being.

Conclusion

In the realm of nutrition, the Keto Vegan diet emerges as a powerful fusion of health and compassion. It transcends boundaries, offering a symphony of vibrant plant-based foods while embracing the metabolic benefits of ketosis. Through this harmonious blend, individuals like Sarah, Emily, and Olivia have witnessed transformative changes: heightened energy, weight loss, radiant skin, and improved heart health. It's a testament to the incredible potential of mindful eating. As this lifestyle gains momentum, it promises not only individual well-being but also a brighter, sustainable future for our planet. The Keto Vegan diet is more than a regimen; it's a celebration of vitality, kindness, and holistic health. Enjoy your meal! It's important to note that while the Keto Vegan Diet offers a range of potential health benefits, it may not be suitable for everyone. It is advisable to consult a healthcare professional or registered dietitian before embarking on this dietary changes, especially if you have underlying health conditions or specific nutritional needs.

4 Weeks Meal Plan

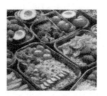

Week 1:

Day 1:
Breakfast: Scrambled Tofu with Spinach and Cherry Tomatoes
Ingredients: Firm tofu, spinach, cherry tomatoes, olive oil, nutritional yeast
Lunch: Zucchini Noodles with Avocado Pesto
Ingredients: Zucchini, avocado, basil, lemon juice, pine nuts
Dinner: Baked Portobello Mushrooms with Garlic Butter Sauce
Ingredients: Portobello mushrooms, coconut oil, garlic, parsley, nutritional yeast
Snack: Almonds and Sliced Cucumber
Day 2:
Breakfast: Chia Seed Pudding with Almond Butter and Berries
Ingredients: Chia seeds, almond butter, unsweetened almond milk, berries, stevia (optional)
Lunch: Cauliflower and Broccoli Salad with Lemon Tahini Dressing
Ingredients: Cauliflower, broccoli, tahini, lemon juice, sesame seeds
Dinner: Stir-Fried Tofu with Bok Choy and Tamari Sauce
Ingredients: Tofu, bok choy, tamari, sesame oil, green onions
Snack: Celery Sticks with Peanut Butter
Day 3:
Breakfast: Almond Flour Pancakes with Coconut Yogurt and Berries
Ingredients: Almond flour, coconut yogurt, berries, baking powder, almond extract
Lunch: Spinach and Avocado Salad with Lemon Vinaigrette
Ingredients: Spinach, avocado, lemon juice, olive oil, sunflower seeds
Dinner: Stuffed Bell Peppers with Cauliflower Rice and Black Beans
Ingredients: Bell peppers, cauliflower rice, black beans, tomato sauce, cumin
Snack: Sliced Bell Peppers with Guacamole
Day 4:
Breakfast: Green Smoothie with Spinach, Avocado, and Coconut Milk
Ingredients: Spinach, avocado, coconut milk, chia seeds, stevia (optional)
Lunch: Tomato and Cucumber Salad with Olive Oil and Herbs
Ingredients: Tomatoes, cucumber, olive oil, fresh herbs (e.g., basil, parsley), salt
Dinner: Eggplant and Zucchini Skewers with Pesto
Ingredients: Eggplant, zucchini, basil pesto (made with basil, pine nuts, olive oil, garlic)
Snack: Cherry Tomatoes and Olives
Day 5:
Breakfast: Coconut Yogurt Parfait with Almonds and Berries
Ingredients: Coconut yogurt, almonds, berries, stevia (optional)

Lunch: Spinach and Mushroom Saute with Garlic and Olive Oil
Ingredients: Spinach, mushrooms, garlic, olive oil, lemon juice
Dinner: Vegan Caesar Salad with Crispy Tofu Croutons
Ingredients: Romaine lettuce, tofu, vegan Caesar dressing, nutritional yeast, olive oil
Snack: Avocado Slices with Sea Salt
Day 6:
Breakfast: Kale and Avocado Smoothie
Ingredients: Kale, avocado, coconut milk, chia seeds, stevia (optional)
Lunch: Cauliflower Rice Stir-Fry with Tofu
Ingredients: Cauliflower rice, tofu, bell peppers, coconut aminos, sesame oil
Dinner: Zucchini Noodles with Pesto and Cherry Tomatoes
Ingredients: Zucchini, basil pesto, cherry tomatoes, olive oil, nutritional yeast
Snack: Cucumber Slices with Hummus
Day 7:
Breakfast: Coconut Flour Pancakes with Almond Butter
Ingredients: Coconut flour, almond butter, almond milk, flaxseed meal, stevia
(optional)
Lunch: Broccoli and Mushroom Salad with Lemon Tahini Dressing
Ingredients: Broccoli, mushrooms, tahini, lemon juice, hemp seeds
Dinner: Spaghetti Squash with Vegan Alfredo Sauce
Ingredients: Spaghetti squash, cashews, nutritional yeast, garlic, almond milk
Snack: Sliced Bell Peppers with Guacamole

Week2:

Day 1:
Breakfast: Blueberry Chia Pudding
Ingredients: Chia seeds, coconut milk, blueberries, vanilla extract, stevia (optional)
Lunch: Spinach and Avocado Salad with Balsamic Vinaigrette
Ingredients: Spinach, avocado, balsamic vinegar, olive oil, pine nuts
Dinner: Stuffed Bell Peppers with Lentils and Tomato Sauce
Ingredients: Bell peppers, green lentils, tomato sauce, garlic, Italian seasoning
Snack: Sliced Radishes with Dairy-Free Ranch Dressing
Day 2:
Breakfast: Chocolate Almond Butter Smoothie
Ingredients: Spinach, almond butter, unsweetened almond milk, cacao powder,
stevia (optional)
Lunch: Cabbage and Carrot Slaw with Creamy Dijon Dressing
Ingredients: Cabbage, carrots, vegan mayo, Dijon mustard, apple cider vinegar
Dinner: Portobello Mushroom Steaks with Garlic Butter
Ingredients: Portobello mushrooms, coconut oil, garlic, parsley, nutritional yeast
Snack: Celery Sticks with Peanut Butter
Day 3:
Breakfast: Chia Seed Pudding with Mixed Berries
Ingredients: Chia seeds, mixed berries, coconut milk, vanilla extract, stevia
(optional)
Lunch: Asparagus and Tomato Salad with Lemon Herb Dressing

Ingredients: Asparagus, tomatoes, lemon juice, fresh herbs (e.g., basil, parsley), olive oil
Dinner: Cauliflower and Broccoli Bake with Vegan Cheese
Ingredients: Cauliflower, broccoli, vegan cheese, almond milk, smoked paprika
Snack: Sliced Radishes with Dairy-Free Ranch Dressing
Day 4:
Breakfast: Avocado and Tomato Toast
Ingredients: Whole grain bread, avocado, tomatoes, olive oil, salt
Lunch: Mushroom and Spinach Saute with Garlic
Ingredients: Mushrooms, spinach, garlic, olive oil, lemon juice
Dinner: Eggplant and Zucchini Skewers with Pesto
Ingredients: Eggplant, zucchini, basil pesto (made with basil, pine nuts, olive oil, garlic)
Snack: Almonds and Cherry Tomatoes
Day 5:
Breakfast: Coconut Yogurt Parfait with Almonds and Berries
Ingredients: Coconut yogurt, almonds, berries, stevia (optional)
Lunch: Lentil and Tomato Salad with Balsamic Dressing
Ingredients: Green lentils, tomatoes, balsamic vinegar, olive oil, fresh herbs (e.g., basil, parsley)
Dinner: Stuffed Bell Peppers with Cauliflower Rice and Black Beans
Ingredients: Bell peppers, cauliflower rice, black beans, tomato sauce, cumin
Snack: Sliced Avocado with Sea Salt
Day 6:
Breakfast: Avocado and Spinach Smoothie (avocado, spinach, almond milk, chia seeds, stevia)
Lunch: Zucchini Noodles with Pesto (zucchini noodles, vegan pesto sauce, cherry tomatoes, pine nuts)
Dinner: Cauliflower Steaks with Vegan Cheese Sauce (cauliflower steaks, nutritional yeast, almond milk, olive oil)
Snack: Cucumber Slices with Guacamole
Day 7:
Breakfast: Chia Pudding with Berries (chia seeds, coconut milk, berries, stevia)
Lunch: Vegan Keto Salad (mixed greens, avocado, cucumber, tofu, olive oil, lemon juice)
Dinner: Eggplant and Mushroom Stir-Fry with Cauliflower Rice (eggplant, mushrooms, cauliflower rice, tamari sauce)
Snack: Almonds and Brazil Nuts

Week 3

Day 1:
Breakfast: Coconut Yogurt Parfait (coconut yogurt, raspberries, unsweetened shredded coconut, chia seeds)
Lunch: Avocado and Cabbage Wraps with Spicy Tahini Sauce (avocado, cabbage leaves, tahini, hot sauce)

Dinner: Spaghetti Squash with Vegan Alfredo Sauce (spaghetti squash, cashews, nutritional yeast, garlic)

Snack: Celery Sticks with Almond Butter

Day 2:

Breakfast: Almond Flour Pancakes with Sugar-Free Syrup (almond flour, flaxseed meal, almond milk, erythritol)

Lunch: Stuffed Bell Peppers with Tofu and Spinach (bell peppers, tofu, spinach, nutritional yeast)

Dinner: Portobello Mushrooms with Garlic and Thyme (portobello mushrooms, garlic, thyme, olive oil)

Snack: Coconut Chips

Day 3:

Breakfast: Vegan Breakfast Burrito (coconut flour tortilla, tofu scramble, avocado, salsa)

Lunch: Cabbage and Avocado Salad with Lemon-Tahini Dressing (cabbage, avocado, tahini, lemon juice)

Dinner: Broccoli and Vegan Cheese Soup (broccoli, nutritional yeast, almond milk)

Snack: Olives and Pickles

Day 4:

Breakfast: Chia Seed Breakfast Bowl (chia seeds, almond milk, almond butter, cinnamon)

Lunch: Grilled Portobello Mushroom Burgers (portobello mushrooms, lettuce, tomato, avocado, vegan cheese)

Dinner: Vegan Cauliflower Pizza Crust with Vegetables (cauliflower, almond flour, flaxseed meal, tomato sauce, veggies)

Snack: Seaweed Snacks

Day 5:

 Breakfast: Flaxseed and Coconut Flour Waffles (flaxseed meal, coconut flour, almond milk, erythritol)

Lunch: Vegan Caesar Salad with Chickpea Croutons (romaine lettuce, chickpeas, vegan Caesar dressing)

Dinner: Stuffed Bell Peppers with Cauliflower Rice and Black Beans (bell peppers, cauliflower rice, black beans, spices)

Snack: Cucumber Slices with Hummus

Day 6:

Breakfast:

Chia Seed Pudding with Almond Butter and Berries (Chia seeds Almond butter Mixed berries Unsweetened almond milk Stevia (optional))

Lunch:

Cauliflower Rice Stir-Fry with Tofu and Broccoli (Cauliflower rice Firm tofu Broccoli florets Tamari sauce Sesame oil)

Dinner:

Spaghetti Squash with Vegan Pesto and Cherry Tomatoes (Spaghetti squash Basil pesto (vegan) Cherry tomatoes Pine nuts

Snack: Sliced Cucumbers with Avocado Dip (Cucumbers Avocado Lime juice Salt)

Day7:

Breakfast: Vegan Scrambled Tofu with Spinach and Mushrooms (Extra-firm tofu Spinach Mushrooms Turmeric Nutritional yeast)
Lunch: Vegan Keto Salad with Avocado, Radishes, and Hemp Seeds (Mixed greens Avocado Radishes Hemp seeds Olive oil)
Dinner: Baked Portobello Mushrooms with Vegan Cheese and Spinach (Portobello mushrooms Vegan cheese Spinach Garlic Olive oil)
Snack: Mixed Nuts (Almonds, Walnuts, Pecans)

Week 4

Day 1:
Breakfast: Coconut Yogurt with Chia Seeds, Flaked Coconut, and Almonds Coconut yogurt (unsweetened) Chia seeds Flaked coconut Almonds
Lunch Bell Peppers with Cauliflower Rice and Black Beans (Bell peppers Cauliflower rice Black beans Cumin Paprika)
Dinner: Zucchini Noodles with Vegan Alfredo Sauce and Cherry Tomatoes (Zucchini Cashews Nutritional yeast Garlic Cherry tomatoes)
Snack: Sliced Bell Peppers with Guacamole (Bell peppers Avocado Lime juice Cilantro)
Day2:
Breakfast: Avocado and Zucchini Smoothie (Avocado Zucchini Unsweetened almond milk Chia seeds
Stevia (optional)
Lunch: Stuffed Bell Peppers Bell peppers (Cauliflower rice Black beans Cumin Paprika)
Dinner: Vegan Pesto Zoodles (Zucchini noodles (zoodles) Vegan pesto sauce Pine nuts Nutritional yeast)
Snack: Sliced Bell Peppers with Guacamole (Bell peppers Avocado Lime juice Cilantro)
Day 3:
Breakfast: Almond Flour Pancakes (Almond flour Flaxseed meal Baking powder Unsweetened almond milk Erythritol (or preferred sweetener)
Lunch: Avocado and Arugula Salad (Avocado Arugula Cherry tomatoes Sunflower seeds Olive oil)
Dinner: Spaghetti Squash with Vegan Alfredo (Spaghetti squash Cashews Nutritional yeast Garlic Parsley)
Snack: Seaweed Snacks
Day 4:
Breakfast: Vegan Tofu Scramble with Spinach (Extra-firm tofu Spinach Turmeric Nutritional yeast Garlic powder)
Lunch: Vegan Keto Bowl (Cauliflower rice Tofu Avocado Hemp seeds Tamari sauce)
Dinner: Eggplant and Spinach Curry (Eggplant Spinach Coconut milk Curry powder Ginger) Snack: Celery Sticks with Almond Butter (Celery stick Almond butter)
Day 5:

Breakfast: Chia Seed Breakfast Bowl (Chia seeds Unsweetened almond milk Almond butter Cinnamon Stevia (optional)
Lunch: Vegan Caesar Salad with Chickpea Croutons (Romaine lettuce Chickpeas Nutritional yeast Olive oil Garlic powder)
Dinner: Vegan Cauliflower Pizza (Cauliflower florets Almond flour Flaxseed meal Tomato sauce Vegan cheese)
Snack: Olives and Pickles (Assorted olives Pickles
Day 6:
Breakfast: Flaxseed and Coconut Flour Waffles (Flaxseed meal Coconut flour Unsweetened almond milk Erythritol (or preferred sweetener) Baking powder)
Lunch: Vegan Sushi Rolls (Nori sheets Cauliflower rice Avocado Cucumber Tofu
Dinner: Vegan Creamed Spinach with Garlic (Spinach Coconut milk Garlic Nutritional yeast Olive oil)
Snack: Cabbage Leaves with Spicy Tahini Sauce (Cabbage leaves Tahini Sriracha (or preferred hot sauce) Lemon juice Water)
Day 7:
Breakfast: Coconut Chia Pudding with Almonds (Chia seeds Coconut milk Stevia (optional) Almonds)
Lunch: Vegan Caesar Salad (Romaine lettuce Cherry tomatoes Avocado Vegan Caesar dressing Hemp seeds)
Dinner: Portobello Mushroom Steaks (Portobello mushrooms Balsamic vinegar Olive oil Garlic Thyme)
Snack: Mixed Nuts (Almonds, Walnuts, Pecans)
Note: As always, adjust portion sizes to meet your personal dietary needs and activity levels. Make sure you stay well-hydrated and always feel free to modify the snacks based on your preferences and ingredient availability. Enjoy your keto vegan meals!

Breakfast Recipes

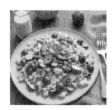

5-Ingredient Vegan Keto Oatmeal

This delightful winter breakfast features a keto vegan oatmeal base, enriched with hemp seeds, flax meal, chia seeds, and psyllium husks, all topped with a sprinkle of cinnamon, turmeric, shredded coconut, and juicy blueberries. This low-carb oatmeal is not only delicious but also packed with fiber, healthy fats, and vegan protein.
Preparation Time: 5 minutes

Cook Time: 2 minutes
Servings: 2

Ingredients:

¼ cup hemp seeds
1 tablespoon flax meal
2 teaspoons chia seeds
1 teaspoon whole psyllium husks (or ½ teaspoon of psyllium husk powder)
⅓ cup coconut milk (unsweetened and full-fat, from a can)
Optional Additions:
1 tablespoon powdered MCT oil
Sprinkle of cinnamon
Sprinkle of turmeric
1 tablespoon shaved coconut
7 blueberries
4 drops liquid stevia
4 drops vanilla extract

Directions:

1. In a medium bowl, combine the hemp seeds, flax meal, chia seeds, psyllium husks, and coconut milk. Let it sit for a minute to thicken.
2. Give it another gentle stir, then microwave for one minute. Remove from the microwave and give it a stir again. If needed, microwave in 20-second intervals, stirring each time, until it's steamy hot.
3. If using, add the MCT powder, stevia, and vanilla extract. Allow it to sit for another minute to reach the desired thickness. If it becomes too thick, add some water to achieve the desired consistency.

Top with cinnamon, turmeric, shaved coconut, and blueberries.

Notes: One bowl serves two.

The optional ingredients is listed in the recipe is included in the nutritional information.

Additionally, you can consider adding other ingredients like pea protein powder, inulin powder, alternative sweeteners, extracts (such as maple syrup extract), and a variety of berries, nut butters, spices, and seeds for added flavor and nutrition.

Nutritional Information (per serving): Calories: 316.5 Fat: 26.6g (41%) Carbohydrates: 9.5g (3%) Protein: 11.5g (23%) Sodium: 7.6mg (0%) Potassium: 111.3mg (3%) Fiber: 5.8g (24%

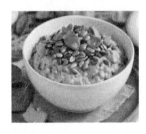

Avocado and Spinach Breakfast Bowl with pumpkin seeds

A nutritious bowl featuring creamy avocado and vibrant spinach, topped with seeds for an extra crunch.

Preparation Time: 10 minutes
Cooking Time: 0 minutes
Total Time: 10 minutes
Serving Size: 1

Ingredients:
1/2 avocado, sliced
1 cup fresh spinach leaves
1 tablespoon pumpkin seeds
1 tablespoon hemp seeds
1 teaspoon lemon juice

Directions:
1. Arrange fresh spinach in a bowl.
2. Top with avocado slices and sprinkle pumpkin seeds and hemp seeds.
3. Drizzle with lemon juice.

*Nutritional Info (per serving): Calories: 227 kcal Protein: 8g (14%) Carbohydrate: 9g (16%) Fat: 18g (70%) Sodium: 20mg Potassium: 741mg Fiber: 7*Coconut Chia Pudding with mixed berries

Creamy chia pudding made with coconut milk and topped with fresh berries.

Preparation Time: 5 minutes (plus overnight chilling)
Cooking Time: 0 minutes
Total Time: 5 minutes (plus overnight chilling)
Serving Size: 1

Ingredients:
2 tablespoons chia seeds
1/2 cup unsweetened coconut milk
1 tablespoon shredded coconut
1/4 cup mixed berries
1 teaspoon erythritol (or sweetener of choice)

Directions:
1. Mix chia seeds and coconut milk in a bowl. Refrigerate overnight.
2. Top with shredded coconut, mixed berries, and sweetener.

Nutritional Info (per serving): Calories: 215 kcal Protein: 5g (15%) Carbohydrate: 16g (24%) Fat: 14g (61%) Sodium: 12mg Potassium: 240mg Fiber: 11g

Almond Butter and Banana Smoothie

A rich and creamy smoothie made with almond butter and ripe bananas.

Preparation Time: 5 minutes
Cooking Time: 0 minutes
Total Time: 5 minutes
Serving Size: 1

Ingredients:
1 tablespoon almond butter

1 ripe banana
1 cup unsweetened almond milk
1 tablespoon chia seeds
1/2 teaspoon vanilla extract
Directions:
1. Blend almond butter, banana, almond milk, chia seeds, and vanilla extract until smooth.
2. Remove from the blender and serve immediately
Nutritional Info (per serving): Calories: 295 kcal Protein: 7g (19%) Carbohydrate: 31g (42%) Fat: 17g (52%) Sodium: 10mg Potassium: 487mg Fiber: 9g

Zucchini and Mushroom Breakfast Scramble

A hearty scramble with zucchini, mushrooms, and tofu, seasoned to perfection.
Preparation Time: 10 minutes
Cooking Time: 10 minutes
Total Time: 20 minutes
Serving Size: 2
Ingredients:
1 medium zucchini, grated
1 cup mushrooms, sliced
1/2 block firm tofu, crumbled
2 tablespoons nutritional yeast
1 tablespoon olive oil
Directions:
1. Heat olive oil in a skillet. Add mushrooms and zucchini. Sauté until tender.
2. Add crumbled tofu and nutritional yeast. Cook until heated through.
Nutritional Info (per serving): Calories: 164 kcal Protein: 14g (20%) Carbohydrate: 8g (10%) Fat: 9g (49%) Sodium: 7mg Potassium: 491mg Fiber: 3g

Chia Seed Breakfast Bowl

A filling bowl packed with chia seeds, nuts, and berries, all soaked in creamy coconut milk.
Preparation Time: 5 minutes (plus overnight soaking)
Cooking Time: 0 minutes
Total Time: 5 minutes (plus overnight soaking)
Serving Size: 1
Ingredients:
2 tablespoons chia seeds
1/2 cup unsweetened coconut milk
1 tablespoon almonds, chopped
1 tablespoon walnuts, chopped
1/4 cup mixed berries
Directions:
1. Mix chia seeds and coconut milk. Refrigerate overnight.
2. Top with chopped almonds, walnuts, and mixed berries.
Nutritional Info (per serving): Calories: 278 kcal Protein: 8g (15%) Carbohydrate: 14g (20%) Fat: 22g (65%) Sodium: 13mg Potassium: 262mg Fiber: 10g

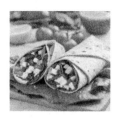

Spinach and Tofu Breakfast Wrap

A protein-packed wrap with sautéed spinach and tofu, wrapped in a low-carb tortilla.
Preparation Time: 10 minutes
Cooking Time: 10 minutes
Total Time: 20 minutes
Serving Size: 1
Ingredients:
2 cups fresh spinach
1/2 block firm tofu, sliced
1 low-carb tortilla
1 tablespoon olive oil
Salt and pepper to taste
Directions:
1. Sauté spinach in olive oil until wilted. Set aside.
2. Cook tofu slices in the same pan until golden on both sides. Season with salt and pepper.
3. Assemble the wrap with spinach and tofu in the tortilla.
Nutritional Info (per serving): Calories: 292 kcal Protein: 22g (30%) Carbohydrate: 13g (18%) Fat: 18g (52%) Sodium: 414mg Potassium: 734mg Fiber: 7g

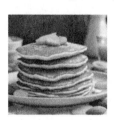

Almond Flour Pancakes

Fluffy pancakes made with almond flour, perfect for a satisfying and low-carb breakfast.
Preparation Time: 10 minutes
Cooking Time: 10 minutes
Total Time: 20 minutes
Serving Size: 2 pancakes
Ingredients:
1 cup almond flour
2 flax eggs (2 tablespoons ground flaxseeds + 6 tablespoons water)

1/4 teaspoon baking powder
1 tablespoon coconut oil
2 tablespoons sugar-free maple syrup
Directions:
1. Mix almond flour, flax eggs, and baking powder in a bowl until well combined.
2. Heat coconut oil on a griddle. Pour batter to make pancakes.
3. Cook until golden on both sides.
4. Serve with sugar-free maple syrup and enjoy
Nutritional Info (per serving, 2 pancakes): Calories: 446 kcal Protein: 13g (12%)
Carbohydrate: 16g (14%) Fat: 39g (74%) Sodium: 21mg Potassium: 170mg Fiber: 8g

Avocado & Chia Pudding

Creamy avocado and chia seeds combine for a satisfying, nutrient-dense pudding.
Preparation Time: 10 minutes
Cooking Time: 0 minutes
Total Time: 10 minutes
Serving Size: 1
Ingredients:
1 medium ripe avocado
2 tbsp chia seeds
1 cup unsweetened almond milk
1 tsp vanilla extract
1 tbsp erythritol (optional, for sweetness)
Directions:
1. Blend avocado, almond milk, vanilla extract, and erythritol (if using) until smooth.
Stir in chia seeds and refrigerate for at least 2 hours or overnight.
Before serving, stir well and add extra almond milk if desired.
Nutritional Info (approximate): Calories: 320 kcal Protein: 7g (9%) Carbohydrate: 15g (5%)
Fat: 27g (76%) Sodium: 40mg Potassium: 975mg Fiber: 12g

Coconut Flour Pancakes

Fluffy and delicious, these pancakes are a keto-friendly twist on a classic.
Preparation Time: 10 minutes
Cooking Time: 10 minutes
Total Time: 20 minutes
Serving Size: 2 pancakes
Ingredients:
1/4 cup coconut flour
2 tbsp ground flaxseed
1 tsp baking powder
1/2 cup unsweetened almond milk
2 tbsp coconut oil (for cooking)
Directions:
1. Mix coconut flour, ground flaxseed, and baking powder in a bowl.
2. Gradually add almond milk and stir until well combined.

3. Heat coconut oil in a non-stick pan. Pour batter to form pancakes.
4. Cook until edges are golden brown, then flip and cook the other side.
Nutritional Info (per serving): Calories: 270 kcal Protein: 9g (15%) Carbohydrate: 14g (7%) Fat: 20g (67%) Sodium: 560mg Potassium: 240mgFiber: 9g

Flaxseed & Spinach Muffins

These savory muffins are loaded with healthy fats and fiber.
Preparation Time: 15 minutes
Cooking Time: 25 minutes
Total Time: 40 minutes
Serving Size: 1 muffin
Ingredients:
1/2 cup ground flaxseed
1/4 cup coconut flour
1 tsp baking powder
1/2 cup unsweetened almond milk
1 cup chopped spinach
Directions:
1. Preheat oven to 350°F (175°C). Line a muffin tin with paper liners.
2. Combine flaxseed, coconut flour, and baking powder in a bowl.
3. Add almond milk and mix until a batter forms. Fold in chopped spinach.
4. Divide the batter into muffin cups and bake for 25 minutes.
Nutritional Info (per serving): Calories: 160 kcal Protein: 6g (15%) Carbohydrate: 9g (5%) Fat: 11g (78%) Sodium: 50mg Potassium: 330mg Fiber: 8g

Mushroom & Spinach Tofu Scramble

A hearty and savory tofu scramble with nutritious veggies.
Preparation Time: 10 minutes
Cooking Time: 10 minutes
Total Time: 20 minutes
Serving Size: 1
Ingredients:
1/2 block firm tofu, crumbled
1 cup sliced mushrooms
1 cup chopped spinach
2 tbsp coconut oil
1/2 tsp turmeric (for color)
Directions:
1. Heat coconut oil in a pan. Add mushrooms and cook until tender.
2. Add crumbled tofu and turmeric. Stir until tofu is evenly coated.
3. Add spinach and cook until wilted.
Nutritional Info (approximate): Calories: 360 kcal Protein: 25g (20%) Carbohydrate: 8g (5%) Fat: 25g (63%) Sodium: 60mg Potassium: 705mg Fiber: 3g

Cauliflower Hash Browns with almond flour

Crispy hash browns made from cauliflower, a low-carb alternative to the classic.
Preparation Time: 15 minutes
Cooking Time: 15 minutes
Total Time: 30 minutes
Serving Size: 4
Ingredients:
3 cups cauliflower florets
1/4 cup almond flour
2 tablespoons olive oil
Salt and pepper to taste
2 tablespoons nutritional yeast
Directions:
1. Pulse cauliflower in a food processor until it reaches a rice-like texture.
2. Mix cauliflower, almond flour, and nutritional yeast. Form batter into patties.
3. Fry in the heated olive oil until golden on both sides. Remove from the heat and serve. Enjoy!
Nutritional Info (per serving): Calories: 132 kcal Protein: 5g (15%) Carbohydrate: 8g (9%) Fat: 10g (67%) Sodium: 34mg Potassium: 377mg Fiber: 4g

Vegan Tofu Scramble

A savory scramble made with tofu and a blend of spices for a satisfying and protein-rich breakfast.
Preparation Time: 10 minutes
Cooking Time: 10 minutes
Total Time: 20 minutes
Serving Size: 2
Ingredients:
1 block firm tofu, crumbled
2 tablespoons nutritional yeast
1 teaspoon turmeric powder
1 tablespoon olive oil
Salt and pepper to taste
Directions:
1. Heat olive oil in a pan.
2. Add crumbled tofu, nutritional yeast, turmeric, salt, and pepper.
3. Cook until heated through.
4. Remove from the heat and serve immediately
Nutritional Info (per serving): Calories: 165 kcal Protein: 16g (20%) Carbohydrate: 5g (10%) Fat: 10g (55%) Sodium: 12mg Potassium: 344mg Fiber: 2g

Flaxseed and Coconut Porridge

A warm and hearty porridge made from flaxseeds and coconut milk, perfect for a cozy breakfast.
Preparation Time: 5 minutes
Cooking Time: 10 minutes
Total Time: 15 minutes

Serving Size: 2
Ingredients:
1/2 cup ground flaxseeds
1 1/2 cups unsweetened coconut milk
2 tablespoons shredded coconut
1 tablespoon erythritol (or sweetener of choice)
1/4 teaspoon cinnamon
Directions:
1. Combine ground flaxseeds, coconut milk, and cinnamon in a pot. Cook over medium heat until thickened.
2. Serve topped with shredded coconut and sweetener.
Nutritional Info (per serving): Calories: 278 kcal Protein: 8g (12%) Carbohydrate: 13g (18%) Fat: 24g (70%) Sodium: 32mg Potassium: 452mg Fiber: 10g

Lunch Recipes

Cauliflower Fried Rice with tofu

This keto-friendly vegan lunch is a low-carb twist on a classic. Cauliflower rice is sautéed with colorful veggies and tofu for a satisfying and nutritious meal.
Preparation Time: 15 minutes
Cooking Time: 15 minutes
Total Time: 30 minutes
Serving Size: 2
Ingredients:
1 medium cauliflower, grated
1 cup tofu, cubed
1 cup mixed vegetables (e.g., bell peppers, broccoli, and carrots)
2 cloves garlic, minced
2 tablespoons tamari sauce
Directions:
1. Heat a large skillet or wok over medium heat. Add a bit of oil.
2. Sauté garlic until fragrant, then add tofu and cook until golden.
3. Add mixed vegetables and stir-fry until tender-crisp.
4. Add grated cauliflower and tamari sauce. Cook for another 5-7 minutes.
5. Serve hot.
Nutritional Information (per serving): Calories: 250 Protein: 15g Carbohydrates: 15g Fat: 16g Sodium: 680mg Potassium: 720mg Fiber: 8g

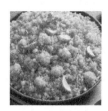

Avocado Zoodle Bowl

This refreshing zoodle bowl features spiralized zucchini, creamy avocado, and a tangy lime dressing. It's a light and energizing keto vegan lunch option.
Preparation Time: 15 minutes
Cooking Time: 0 minutes
Total Time: 15 minutes
Serving Size: 2
Ingredients:
2 medium zucchinis, spiralized
2 avocados, sliced
1 cup cherry tomatoes, halved
1/4 cup fresh cilantro, chopped
2 tablespoons lime juice
Directions:
1. Arrange zucchini noodles, avocado slices, and cherry tomatoes in a bowl.
2. Drizzle with lime juice and garnish with cilantro.
Nutritional Information (per serving): Calories: 310 Protein: 6g Carbohydrates: 18g Fat: 26g Sodium: 10mg Potassium: 1050mg Fiber: 12g

Creamy Coconut and Spinach Soup

This rich, velvety soup combines the goodness of coconut and nutrient-dense spinach.
Preparation Time: 10 minutes
Cooking Time: 15 minutes
Total Time: 25 minutes
Serving Size: 2
Ingredients:
1 can (400ml) full-fat coconut milk
2 cups fresh spinach leaves
2 cloves garlic, minced
1 tbsp coconut oil
Salt and pepper to taste
Directions:
1. In a pot, heat coconut oil and sauté minced garlic until fragrant.
2. Add coconut milk and bring to a gentle simmer.
3. Stir in fresh spinach and cook until wilted.
4. Blend the mixture until smooth. Season with salt and pepper.
Nutritional Info (per serving): Calories: 380 kcal Protein: 6g (16%) Carbohydrate: 7g (8%) Fat: 38g (76%) Sodium: 30mg Potassium: 530mg Fiber: 2g

Avocado and Zucchini Noodles

A refreshing noodle dish with creamy avocado sauce and crisp zucchini.
Preparation Time: 15 minutes
Cooking Time: 0 minutes
Total Time: 15 minutes
Serving Size: 2
Ingredients:
2 medium zucchinis, spiralized
2 ripe avocados
2 tbsp olive oil
Juice of 1 lemon
Salt and pepper to taste
Directions:
1. In a bowl, mash avocados and mix with lemon juice, olive oil, salt, and pepper.
2. Toss zucchini noodles in the avocado mixture until well-coated.
Nutritional Info (per serving): Calories: 380 kcal Protein: 6g (16%) Carbohydrate: 18g (10%) Fat: 32g (76%) Sodium: 20mg Potassium: 1080mg Fiber: 12g

Cauliflower and Walnut Salad

A crunchy salad packed with healthy fats and nutrients.
Preparation Time: 10 minutes
Cooking Time: 10 minutes
Total Time: 20 minutes
Serving Size: 2
Ingredients:
2 cups cauliflower florets, steamed
1/2 cup walnuts, chopped
1/4 cup olive oil
2 tbsp lemon juice
Salt and pepper to taste
Directions:
1. In a bowl, combine steamed cauliflower and chopped walnuts.
2. Drizzle olive oil and lemon juice. Season with salt and pepper. Toss to combine. Enjoy!
Nutritional Info (per serving): Calories: 400 kcal Protein: 7g (16%) Carbohydrate: 10g (8%) Fat: 38g (76%) Sodium: 30mg Potassium: 590mg Fiber: 4g

Mushroom and Spinach Stuffed Bell Peppers

These stuffed peppers are hearty, flavorful, and loaded with nutritious veggies.
Preparation Time: 20 minutes
Cooking Time: 25 minutes
Total Time: 45 minutes
Serving Size: 2
Ingredients:
2 large bell peppers

1 cup mushrooms, chopped
2 cups fresh spinach
2 tbsp olive oil
Salt and pepper to taste

Directions:

1. Preheat oven to 375°F (190°C). Cut the tops off the bell peppers and remove seeds.
2. In a pan, sauté mushrooms and spinach in olive oil until tender. Season with salt and pepper.
3. Stuff the peppers with the mushroom and spinach mixture. Bake for 25 minutes.
4. Remove from the heat and serve.Enjoy!

Nutritional Info (per serving): Calories: 350 kcal Protein: 7g (16%) Carbohydrate: 16g (10%) Fat: 30g (76%) Sodium: 40mg Potassium: 940mg Fiber: 6g

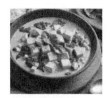

Coconut and Almond Tofu Stir-Fry

A quick and satisfying stir-fry with a creamy coconut and almond sauce.
Preparation Time: 15 minutes
Cooking Time: 15 minutes
Total Time: 30 minutes
Serving Size: 2
Ingredients:
1 block firm tofu, cubed
1/2 cup coconut milk
1/4 cup almond butter
2 tbsp coconut oil
2 cups mixed vegetables (broccoli, bell peppers, snap peas)
Directions:
1. In a wok or large skillet, heat coconut oil and add cubed tofu. Cook until golden.
2. Add mixed vegetables and sauté until crisp-tender.
3. In a bowl, whisk coconut milk and almond butter. Pour over the tofu and vegetables.
Nutritional Info (per serving): Calories: 420 kcal Protein: 18g (17%) Carbohydrate: 12g (8%) Fat: 36g (76%) Sodium: 40mg Potassium: 750mg Fiber: 6g

Almond Butter Tofu Stir Fry

This hearty stir fry combines tofu, broccoli, and bell peppers in a rich almond butter sauce. It's a protein-packed keto vegan lunch that will keep you satisfied.
Preparation Time: 20 minutes
Cooking Time: 15 minutes
Total Time: 35 minutes
Serving Size: 2
Ingredients:
1 block extra firm tofu, cubed
1 cup broccoli florets
1 red bell pepper, sliced
2 tablespoons almond butter
2 tablespoons tamari sauce
Directions:
1. Press tofu to remove excess moisture, then sauté until golden in a large skillet.
2. Add broccoli and bell pepper. Cook until vegetables are tender-crisp.
3. In a small bowl, whisk together almond butter and tamari sauce. Pour over the tofu and vegetables.
Stir well and cook for an additional 2-3 minutes.

Nutritional Information (per serving): Calories: 360 Protein: 28g Carbohydrates: 14g Fat: 24g Sodium: 890mg Potassium: 590mg Fiber: 6g

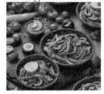

Portobello Mushroom Fajitas

These fajitas feature juicy portobello mushrooms marinated in a zesty blend of spices. They're served with a colorful array of bell peppers and onions for a flavorful keto vegan lunch.
Preparation Time: 20 minutes
Cooking Time: 15 minutes
Total Time: 35 minutes
Serving Size: 2
Ingredients:
4 large portobello mushrooms, sliced
2 bell peppers, thinly sliced
1 large onion, thinly sliced
2 tablespoons olive oil
2 teaspoons chili powder
Directions:
1. In a large bowl, combine mushrooms, bell peppers, onions, olive oil, and chili powder. Toss to coat evenly.
2. Heat a skillet over medium-high heat and add the mushroom mixture.
3. Cook for 10-12 minutes, stirring occasionally, until vegetables are tender. Enjoy!
Nutritional Information (per serving): Calories: 280 Protein: 8g Carbohydrates: 22g Fat: 20g Sodium: 20mg Potassium: 1030mg Fiber: 7g

Spinach and Avocado Salad

This simple salad combines fresh spinach leaves with creamy avocado, cherry tomatoes, and a zesty lemon dressing. It's a light yet satisfying keto vegan lunch option.
Preparation Time: 10 minutes
Cooking Time: 0 minutes
Total Time: 10 minutes
Serving Size: 2
Ingredients:
4 cups fresh spinach leaves
2 avocados, sliced
1 cup cherry tomatoes, halved
2 tablespoons lemon juice
2 tablespoons olive oil
Directions:
1. In a large bowl, combine spinach, avocado, and cherry tomatoes.
2. Drizzle with olive oil and lemon juice.

3. Toss gently to coat.
Nutritional Information (per serving): Calories: 320 Protein: 6g Carbohydrates: 19g Fat: 28g Sodium: 30mg Potassium: 1080mg Fiber: 12g

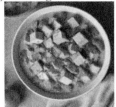

Coconut Curry Tofu

This creamy coconut curry tofu is packed with flavor and spices. It's a comforting and satisfying keto vegan lunch option.
Preparation Time: 15 minutes
Cooking Time: 25 minutes
Total Time: 40 minutes
Serving Size: 2
Ingredients:
1 block extra firm tofu, cubed
1 can coconut milk
2 tablespoons curry powder
1 tablespoon ginger, minced
1 tablespoon garlic, minced
Directions:
1. Press tofu and cut into cubes. Sauté in a large cooking pan until golden brown. Set aside.
2. In the same pan, add coconut milk, curry powder, ginger, and garlic. Simmer for 15-20 minutes.
3. Add the tofu back into the pan and cook for an additional 5 minutes.
Nutritional Information (per serving): Calories: 450 Protein: 21g Carbohydrates: 14g Fat: 38g Sodium: 20mg Potassium: 660mg Fiber: 4g

Avocado Zoodle Salad

This refreshing salad combines zucchini noodles with creamy avocado and a tangy vinaigrette for a satisfying keto vegan lunch.
Preparation Time: 15 minutes
Cooking Time: 0 minutes
Total Time: 15 minutes
Serving Size: 2
Ingredients:
2 medium zucchinis, spiralized
2 ripe avocados, diced
1 cup cherry tomatoes, halved
1/4 cup fresh basil leaves, chopped
2 tablespoons olive oil

2 tablespoons lemon juice
Salt and pepper to taste
Directions:
In a large mixing bowl, combine zucchini noodles, diced avocados, cherry tomatoes, and chopped basil.
Drizzle olive oil and lemon juice over the salad. Season with salt and pepper. Gently toss the ingredients to coat everything evenly.
Serve chilled.
Nutritional Info (per serving): Calories: 390 Protein: 7g (18%) Carbohydrates: 18g (8%) Fat: 35g (74%) Sodium: 150mg Potassium: 1260mg Fiber: 13g

Cauliflower and Chickpea Curry

This flavorful curry combines cauliflower and chickpeas in a creamy coconut sauce for a satisfying keto vegan meal.
Preparation Time: 20 minutes
Cooking Time: 25 minutes
Total Time: 45 minutes
Serving Size: 4
Ingredients:
1 medium cauliflower, cut into florets
1 can (15 oz) chickpeas, drained and rinsed
1 can (15 oz) coconut milk
2 tablespoons curry powder
1 tablespoon coconut oil
Salt to taste
Directions:
1. In a large skillet, heat coconut oil over medium heat. Add cauliflower florets and sauté for 5 minutes.
2. Add chickpeas and curry powder to the skillet. Cook for another 2 minutes.
3. Pour the coconut milk to the pot and bring to a gentle simmer. Cover and cook for 15-20 minutes or until cauliflower is tender.
4. Season with salt to taste. Serve hot.
Nutritional Info (per serving): Calories: 320 Protein: 8g (20%) Carbohydrates: 16g (7%) Fat: 27g (76%) Sodium: 250mg Potassium: 820mg Fiber: 7g

Creamy Spinach and Coconut Soup

This velvety soup combines the richness of coconut milk with the earthy flavor of spinach for a comforting keto vegan lunch.
Preparation Time: 10 minutes
Cooking Time: 20 minutes
Total Time: 30 minutes
Serving Size: 4
Ingredients:
1 lb fresh spinach
1 can (14 oz) coconut milk
1 small onion, chopped

2 cloves garlic, minced
2 tablespoons coconut oil
Salt and pepper to taste
Directions:
1. In a large cooking pot, heat coconut oil over medium heat. Add chopped onion and sauté for a minute to 2 minutes or until translucent.
2. Add minced garlic and cook for another minute until fragrant.
3. Add the fresh spinach and sauté for a minute or until wilted.
4. Pour the coconut milk to the cooking pot and let it simmer for about 15 minutes.
5. Blend the soup with immersion blender until smooth and then Season with salt and pepper to taste.
5. Remove from heat and serve hot.
Nutritional Info (per serving): Calories: 240 Protein: 5g (17%) Carbohydrates: 7g (8%) Fat: 22g (75%) Sodium: 110mg Potassium: 1150mg Fiber: 4g

Spaghetti Squash with Pesto

This dish features roasted spaghetti squash topped with a vibrant basil pesto for a light yet satisfying keto vegan lunch.
Preparation Time: 15 minutes
Cooking Time: 40 minutes
Total Time: 55 minutes
Serving Size: 2
Ingredients:
1 medium spaghetti squash
1 cup fresh basil leaves
1/2 cup pine nuts
1/4 cup olive oil
2 cloves garlic
Salt to taste
Directions:
1. Preheat the oven to 375°F (190°C).
2. Cut the spaghetti squash in half lengthwise and scoop out the seeds. let the halves face down on a baking sheet. Bake for about 40 minutes, or until the flesh is easily pierced with a fork.
3. While the squash is roasting, prepare the pesto. In a food processor, combine basil leaves, pine nuts, garlic, and olive oil. Blend until smooth. Season with salt to taste.
4. Once the squash is cooked, use a fork to scrape out the strands.
5. Toss the spaghetti squash with the pesto until well-coated.
6. Serve warm.
Nutritional Info (per serving): Calories: 360 Protein: 7g (19%) Carbohydrates: 18g (6%) Fat: 30g (75%) Sodium: 140mg Potassium: 660mg Fiber: 5g

Salad Recipes

Simple Spinach and Avocado Salad

A light and refreshing salad featuring fresh spinach leaves and creamy avocado slices.
Preparation Time: 10 minutes
Cooking Time: 0 minutes
Total Time: 10 minutes
Serving Size: 2
Ingredients:
4 cups fresh spinach leaves
1 large avocado, sliced
2 tablespoons olive oil
1 tablespoon lemon juice
Salt and pepper to taste
Directions:
1. In a large bowl, combine the fresh spinach leaves and avocado slices.
2. Drizzle olive oil and lemon juice over the salad.
3. Season with salt and pepper to taste.
4. Gently toss to combine.
5. Serve immediately.
Nutritional Info: Calories: 250 Protein: 10% Carbohydrate: 8% Fat: 82% Sodium: 200mg Potassium: 850mg Fiber: 8g

Zucchini Noodle Salad with Pesto

A vibrant salad featuring fresh zucchini noodles tossed in a flavorful vegan pesto.
Preparation Time: 15 minutes
Cooking Time: 5 minutes
Total Time: 20 minutes
Serving Size: 2
Ingredients:
2 medium zucchinis, spiralized into noodles
1/4 cup vegan pesto sauce
1/4 cup cherry tomatoes, halved
2 tablespoons pine nuts
1/4 cup nutritional yeast (optional, for added flavor)
Directions:
1. In a large mixing bowl, combine zucchini noodles, cherry tomatoes, and pine nuts.
2. Add the vegan pesto sauce and toss until the noodles are evenly coated.
3. If using, sprinkle nutritional yeast over the salad and gently mix.

4. Serve chilled.
Nutritional Info: *Calories: 280 Protein: 17% Carbohydrate: 7% Fat: 76% Sodium: 150mg Potassium: 750mg Fiber: 5g*

Cabbage and Almond Slaw

A crunchy slaw made with shredded cabbage and toasted almonds, dressed in a zesty vinaigrette.
Preparation Time: 15 minutes
Cooking Time: 5 minutes
Total Time: 20 minutes
Serving Size: 4
Ingredients:
4 cups shredded cabbage
1/2 cup sliced almonds, toasted
1/4 cup olive oil
2 tablespoons apple cider vinegar
1 teaspoon Dijon mustard
Salt and pepper to taste
Directions:
1. In a large bowl, combine shredded cabbage and toasted almonds.
2. In a small bowl, whisk together olive oil, apple cider vinegar, Dijon mustard, salt, and pepper.
3. Pour the dressing over the salad and toss until well coated.
4. Serve immediately.
Nutritional Info: Calories: 190nProtein: 18% Carbohydrate: 8% Fat: 74% Sodium: 50mg Potassium: 350mg Fiber: 5g

Cucumber and Radish Salad with Mint

A crisp and refreshing salad with cucumbers, radishes, and fresh mint leaves in a zingy lemon dressing.
Preparation Time: 10 minutes
Cooking Time: 0 minutes
Total Time: 10 minutes
Serving Size: 2
Ingredients:
2 cucumbers, thinly sliced
1 cup radishes, thinly sliced
2 tablespoons fresh mint leaves, chopped
2 tablespoons lemon juice
2 tablespoons olive oil
Salt and pepper to taste
Directions:
1. In a large bowl, combine sliced cucumbers, radishes, and chopped mint leaves.
2. In a small mixing bowl, whisk together olive oil, lemon juice, salt, and pepper.
3. Pour the dressing over the salad and gently toss to combine.
4. Serve salad immediately and enjoy.

Nutritional Info: Calories: 160 Protein: 10% Carbohydrate: 10% Fat: 80% Sodium: 15mgPotassium: 620mg Fiber: 4g

Asparagus and Avocado Salad

A vibrant salad featuring tender asparagus spears and creamy avocado slices in a zesty lemon **dressing.**
Preparation Time: 15 minutes
Cooking Time: 5 minutes
Total Time: 20 minutes
Serving Size: 2
Ingredients:
1 bunch asparagus, trimmed and blanched
1 large avocado, sliced
2 tablespoons lemon juice
2 tablespoons olive oil
Salt and pepper to taste
Directions:
1. Arrange the blanched asparagus and avocado slices on a serving platter.
2. In a small mixing bowl, whisk together the lemon juice, olive oil, salt, and pepper.
3. Drizzle the dressing over the salad.
Gently toss to combine.
4. Serve immediately.
Nutritional Info: Calories: 230 Protein: 15% Carbohydrate: 8% Fat: 77% Sodium: 10mgPotassium: 740mg Fiber: 7g

Tomato and Basil Salad with Balsamic Glaze

A classic combination of juicy tomatoes and fresh basil leaves drizzled with a sweet balsamic glaze.
Preparation Time: 10 minutes
Cooking Time: 0 minutes
Total Time: 10 minutes
Serving Size: 2
Ingredients:
2 large tomatoes, sliced
1/2 cup fresh basil leaves
2 tablespoons balsamic glaze
2 tablespoons olive oil
Salt and pepper to taste
Directions:
1. Arrange the tomato slices and fresh basil leaves on a serving platter.
2. Drizzle balsamic glaze and olive oil over the salad.
3. Season with salt and pepper to taste.
4. Serve immediately and enjoy.
Nutritional Info: Calories: 160 Protein: 10% Carbohydrate: 15% Fat: 75% Sodium: 20mg Potassium: 640mg Fiber: 4g

Kale and Walnut Salad with Lemon Tahini Dressing

A hearty salad featuring nutrient-rich kale and crunchy walnuts, topped with a zesty lemon tahini dressing.

Preparation Time: 15 minutes
Cooking Time: 0 minutes
Total Time: 15 minutes
Serving Size: 2

Ingredients:

4 cups kale leaves, destemmed and chopped
1/2 cup walnuts, roughly chopped
2 tablespoons tahini
2 tablespoons lemon juice
2 tablespoons water
Salt and pepper to taste

Directions:

1. In a large bowl, combine chopped kale leaves and chopped walnuts.
2. In a small bowl, whisk together tahini, lemon juice, water, salt, and pepper.
3. Drizzle the dressing over the salad and toss until well coated.

Divide the salad among to 2 serving plates and Serve immediately.

Nutritional Info: Calories: 260 Protein: 12% Carbohydrate: 10% Fat: 78% Sodium: 40mg Potassium: 700mg Fiber: 6g

Broccoli and Almond Salad with Dijon Vinaigrette

A crunchy salad featuring blanched broccoli florets and toasted almonds, dressed in a tangy Dijon mustard vinaigrette.

Preparation Time: 15 minutes
Cooking Time: 5 minutes
Total Time: 20 minutes
Serving Size: 2

Ingredients:

2 cups broccoli florets, blanched
1/4 cup sliced almonds, toasted
2 tablespoons olive oil
1 tablespoon Dijon mustard
2 tablespoons apple cider vinegar
Salt and pepper to taste

Directions:

1. In a large bowl, combine blanched broccoli florets and toasted almonds.
2. In a small bowl, whisk together olive oil, Dijon mustard, apple cider vinegar, salt, and pepper.

3Pour the dressing over the salad and gently toss to coaqte.
4. Serve immediately.
Nutritional Info: Calories: 220 Protein: 15% Carbohydrate: 12% Fat: 73% Sodium: 80mg Potassium: 530mg Fiber: 5g

Brussels sprouts and Pecan Salad with Maple Vinaigrette

A flavorful salad featuring roasted Brussels sprouts and crunchy pecans, topped with a sweet maple vinaigrette.

Preparation Time: 20 minutes
Cooking Time: 15 minutes
Total Time: 35 minutes
Serving Size: 2

Ingredients:
2 cups Brussels sprouts, halved
1/2 cup pecans, roughly chopped and toasted
2 tablespoons olive oil
2 tablespoons maple syrup
2 tablespoons apple cider vinegar
Salt and pepper to taste

Directions:
1. Preheat the oven to 400°F (200°C). Toss the halved Brussels sprouts in olive oil, then spread them on a baking sheet. Roast for 15 minutes or until golden brown.
2. In a large bowl, combine roasted Brussels sprouts and toasted pecans.
3. In a small bowl, whisk together maple syrup, apple cider vinegar, salt, and pepper.
4. Drizzle the dressing over the salad and toss until well combined.
5. Serve warm.
Nutritional Info: Calories: 250 Protein: 12% Carbohydrate: 15% Fat: 73% Sodium: 30mg Potassium: 520mg Fiber: 7g

Chickpea and Cauliflower Salad with Lemon Tahini Dressing

A satisfying salad featuring roasted cauliflower florets and hearty chickpeas, drizzled with a zesty lemon tahini dressing.

Preparation Time: 20 minutes
Cooking Time: 25 minutes
Total Time: 45 minutes
Serving Size: 2

Ingredients:

2 cups cauliflower florets
1 cup canned chickpeas, drained and rinsed
2 tablespoons tahini
2 tablespoons lemon juice
2 tablespoons olive oil
Salt and pepper to taste

Directions:

1. Preheat the oven to 425°F (220°C). Toss the cauliflower florets in olive oil, then spread them on a baking sheet. Roast until golden brown, for about 25 minutes.
2. In a large bowl, combine roasted cauliflower florets and chickpeas.
3. In a small bowl, whisk together tahini, lemon juice, olive oil, salt, and pepper.
4. Drizzle the dressing over the salad and toss gently to combine.
5. Divide salad into 2 serving plates and Serve warm.

Nutritional Info: Calories: 280 Protein: 16% Carbohydrate: 13% Fat: 71% Sodium: 180mg Potassium: 630mg Fiber: 8g

Mixed Greens and Avocado Salad with Creamy Garlic Dressing

A delightful salad featuring a medley of mixed greens and creamy avocado slices, topped with a luscious garlic dressing.

Preparation Time: 15 minutes
Cooking Time: 0 minutes
Total Time: 15 minutes
Serving Size: 2

Ingredients:

4 cups mixed salad greens
1 large avocado, sliced
2 tablespoons vegan mayonnaise
1 clove garlic, minced
2 tablespoons lemon juice
Salt and pepper to taste

Directions:

1. In a large bowl, combine mixed salad greens and avocado slices.
2. In a small bowl, whisk together vegan mayonnaise, minced garlic, lemon juice, salt, and pepper.
3. Drizzle the dressing over the salad.

4. Gently toss to combine.

5. Divide among 2 serving plates and serve immediately.

Nutritional Info: Calories: 260 Protein: 12% Carbohydrate: 12% Fat: 76%Sodium: 90mg Potassium: 810mg Fiber: 8g

Spinach and Avocado Salad with Raspberry Vinaigrette

A delightful combination of fresh spinach leaves and creamy avocado, topped with a sweet and tangy raspberry vinaigrette.

Preparation Time: 15 minutes
Cooking Time: 0 minutes
Total Time: 15 minutes
Serving Size: 2

Ingredients:
4 cups fresh spinach leaves
1 large avocado, sliced
1/4 cup raspberries (fresh or frozen)
2 tablespoons olive oil
1 tablespoon balsamic vinegar
Salt and pepper to taste

Directions:
1. In a large bowl, combine fresh spinach leaves and avocado slices.
2. In a small bowl, mash raspberries with a fork and whisk in olive oil, balsamic vinegar, salt, and pepper.
3. Drizzle the raspberry vinaigrette over the salad.
4. Gently toss to combine and serve immediately.

Nutritional Info: *Calories: 250 Protein: 12% Carbohydrate: 13% Fat: 75% Sodium: 90mg Potassium: 860mg Fiber: 10g*

Bell Pepper and Cucumber Salad with Lemon Herb Dressing

A vibrant salad featuring colorful bell peppers and crisp cucumber, dressed in a zesty lemon herb dressing.

Preparation Time: 15 minutes
Cooking Time: 0 minutes
Total Time: 15 minutes
Serving Size: 2

Ingredients:
1 red bell pepper, thinly sliced

1 yellow bell pepper, thinly sliced
1 cucumber, thinly sliced
2 tablespoons lemon juice
2 tablespoons olive oil
1 tablespoon fresh herbs (such as parsley or dill), chopped
Salt and pepper to taste
Directions:
1. In a large bowl, combine sliced bell peppers and cucumber.
2. In a small bowl, whisk together lemon juice, olive oil, fresh herbs, salt, and pepper.
3. Drizzle the dressing over the salad.
4. Gently toss to combine.
5. Serve immediately.
Nutritional Info: Calories: 210 Protein: 10% Carbohydrate: 15% Fat: 75% Sodium: 30mg Potassium: 780mg Fiber: 6g

Arugula and Pomegranate Salad with Balsamic Glaze

A vibrant salad featuring peppery arugula and sweet pomegranate seeds, drizzled with a rich balsamic glaze.
Preparation Time: 10 minutes
Cooking Time: 0 minutes
Total Time: 10 minutes
Serving Size: 2
Ingredients:
4 cups arugula leaves
1/2 cup pomegranate seeds
2 tablespoons balsamic glaze
2 tablespoons olive oil
2 tablespoons pumpkin seeds (optional, for added crunch)
Directions:
1. In a large bowl, combine arugula leaves and pomegranate seeds.
2. Drizzle balsamic glaze and olive oil over the salad.
3. Sprinkle pumpkin seeds over the top for added crunch, If using.
4. Gently toss to combine.
5. Serve immediately.
Nutritional Info: Calories: 230 Protein: 12% Carbohydrate: 13% Fat: 75% Sodium: 20mg Potassium: 480mg Fiber: 6g

Romaine and Avocado Caesar Salad

A classic Caesar salad with a twist, featuring crisp romaine lettuce and creamy avocado, dressed in a vegan Caesar dressing.
Preparation Time: 15 minutes
Cooking Time: 0 minutes
Total Time: 15 minutes
Serving Size: 2
Ingredients:

4 cups romaine lettuce, chopped
1 large avocado, diced
2 tablespoons vegan Caesar dressing
2 tablespoons nutritional yeast (optional, for added flavor)
2 tablespoons croutons (optional, for crunch)
Directions:
1. In a large bowl, combine chopped romaine lettuce and diced avocado.
2. Drizzle vegan Caesar dressing over the salad.
3. Sprinkle nutritional yeast for added flavor and croutons for extra crunch, if using.
4. Gently toss to combine.
5. Serve salad immediately.
Nutritional Info: Calories: 240 Protein: 10% Carbohydrate: 15% Fat: 75% Sodium: 120mg Potassium: 770mg Fiber: 10g

Dinner Recipes

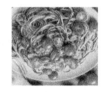

Zucchini Noodles with Pesto and Cherry Tomatoes

Spiralized zucchini noodles tossed with a vibrant basil pesto and fresh cherry tomatoes for a light and flavorful keto vegan dinner.
Preparation Time: 15 minutes
Cooking Time: 0 minutes
Total Time: 15 minutes
Serving Size: 2
Ingredients:
2 medium zucchinis, spiralized
1/2 cup fresh basil leaves
1/4 cup pine nuts
2 tablespoons olive oil
1 cup cherry tomatoes, halved
Directions:
1. In a food processor, combine basil leaves, pine nuts, and olive oil. Blend until smooth.
2. In a large mixing bowl, toss the zucchini noodles with the pesto.
3. Add cherry tomatoes and gently mix.
4. Serve chilled.

Nutritional Info (per serving): Calories: 280 Protein: 6g (20%) Carbohydrates: 10g (7%) Fat: 25g (64%) Sodium: 10mg Potassium: 740mg Fiber: 4g

Portobello Mushroom Steaks

Juicy and flavorful portobello mushrooms marinated and grilled to perfection, served with a side of steamed broccoli.

Preparation Time: 10 minutes
Cooking Time: 10 minutes
Total Time: 20 minutes
Serving Size: 2
Ingredients:
4 large portobello mushroom caps
2 tablespoons balsamic vinegar
2 tablespoons olive oil
4 cloves garlic, minced
1 bunch broccoli, florets separated

Directions:
1. In a small bowl, whisk together balsamic vinegar, olive oil, and minced garlic.
2. Brush the marinade onto both sides of the portobello mushroom caps and let them to marinate for at least 10 minutes.
3. Preheat a grill or grill pan over medium-high heat. Grill the marinated mushrooms for about 5 minutes on each side, or until tender.
4. While the mushrooms are grilling, steam the broccoli florets until tender.
5. Serve the grilled mushrooms with a side of steamed broccoli.
Nutritional Info (per serving): Calories: 320 Protein: 9g (18%) Carbohydrates: 22g (10%) Fat: 24g (68%) Sodium: 50mg Potassium: 1700mg Fiber: 9g

Creamy Coconut Curry with Tofu and Spinach

A luscious coconut-based curry with protein-rich tofu and vibrant spinach.

Preparation Time: 15 minutes
Cooking Time: 20 minutes
Total Time: 35 minutes
Serving Size: 2

Ingredients:
1 block firm tofu, cubed
1 can (400ml) full-fat coconut milk
2 cups fresh spinach leaves
2 tbsp curry powder
2 tbsp coconut oil

Directions:
1. In a large pan, heat coconut oil. Add tofu and cook until golden brown.
2. Add curry powder and stir for a minute. Pour in coconut milk and simmer for 10 minutes.
3. Add fresh spinach and cook until wilted.
Nutritional Info (per serving): Calories: 450 kcal Protein: 15g (13%) Carbohydrate: 10g (9%) Fat: 40g (78%) Sodium: 45mg Potassium: 680mg Fiber: 5g

Mushroom and Avocado Zoodles

A satisfying noodle dish with creamy avocado and earthy mushrooms.
Preparation Time: 15 minutes
Cooking Time: 10 minutes
Total Time: 25 minutes
Serving Size: 2
Ingredients:
2 medium zucchinis, spiralized
2 cups mushrooms, sliced
1 ripe avocado
2 tbsp olive oil
Salt and pepper to taste
Directions:
1. In a large pan, heat olive oil. Sauté mushrooms until golden.
2. In a bowl, mash avocado and season with salt and pepper. Toss with zoodles.
3. Add sautéed mushrooms on top.
Nutritional Info (per serving): Calories: 380 kcal Protein: 8g (17%) Carbohydrate: 14g (10%) Fat: 32g (76%) Sodium: 20mg Potassium: 1120mg Fiber: 10g

Cauliflower and Almond Soup

A creamy, nutty soup with the richness of almonds and cauliflower.
Preparation Time: 10 minutes
Cooking Time: 20 minutes
Total Time: 30 minutes
Serving Size: 2
Ingredients:
2 cups cauliflower florets
1/2 cup almond butter
2 cups vegetable broth
2 tbsp olive oil
Salt and pepper to taste
Directions:
1. Steam cauliflower until tender. Blend with almond butter and vegetable broth until smooth.
2. In a large pot, heat olive oil. Pour in the cauliflower mixture and simmer for 10 minutes.
3. Season with salt and pepper.

Nutritional Info (per serving): Calories: 430 kcal Protein: 12g (11%) Carbohydrate: 12g (10%) Fat: 38g (79%) Sodium: 680mg Potassium: 760mg Fiber: 6g

Stuffed Bell Peppers with Spinach and Pine Nuts

These vibrant peppers are stuffed with hearty spinach and crunchy pine nuts.
Preparation Time: 25 minutes
Cooking Time: 25 minutes
Total Time: 50 minutes
Serving Size: 2

Ingredients:
4 large bell peppers
2 cups fresh spinach leaves
1/4 cup pine nuts
2 tbsp olive oil
Salt and pepper to taste

Directions:
1. Preheat oven to 375°F (190°C). Properly cut off the tops of the bell peppers and remove seeds.
2. In a pan, sauté fresh spinach and pine nuts in olive oil until wilted. Season with salt and pepper.
3. Stuff the peppers with the spinach and pine nut mixture. Bake for 25 minutes.
Nutritional Info (per serving): Calories: 400 kcal Protein: 8g (15%) Carbohydrate: 16g (10%) Fat: 35g (75%) Sodium: 50mg Potassium: 1240mg Fiber: 8g

Creamy Avocado and Asparagus Stir-Fry

A quick and creamy stir-fry featuring avocados and fresh asparagus.
Preparation Time: 15 minutes
Cooking Time: 10 minutes
Total Time: 25 minutes
Serving Size: 2

Ingredients:
1 bunch asparagus, cut into pieces
2 ripe avocados
2 tbsp coconut oil
2 tbsp lemon juice
Salt and pepper to taste

Directions:
1. In a large skillet, heat coconut oil. Add asparagus and cook until crisp-tender.
2. In a bowl, mash avocados with lemon juice, salt, and pepper. Pour over asparagus. Enjoy!

Nutritional Info (per serving): Calories: 420 kcal Protein: 8g (15%) Carbohydrate: 18g (10%) Fat: 38g (75%) Sodium: 20mg Potassium: 1100mg Fiber: 10g

Vegan Cauliflower Alfredo with Spinach

Creamy cauliflower alfredo sauce served over sautéed spinach for a nutritious and satisfying keto vegan dinner.

Preparation Time: 10 minutes
Cooking Time: 20 minutes
Total Time: 30 minutes
Serving Size: 4

Ingredients:
1 medium head cauliflower, chopped
4 cups fresh spinach leaves
1/4 cup nutritional yeast
2 tablespoons olive oil
Salt and pepper to taste

Directions:
1. Steam or boil the cauliflower until tender. Drain and transfer to a blender.
2. Add nutritional yeast, salt, and pepper to the cauliflower in the blender. Blend until smooth and creamy.
3. In a large skillet, heat olive oil over medium heat. Add the spinach and sauté for a minute or until wilted.
4. Serve the cauliflower alfredo sauce over the sautéed spinach.

Nutritional Info (per serving): Calories: 160 Protein: 7g (20%) Carbohydrates: 10g (6%) Fat: 10g (56%) Sodium: 120mg Potassium: 740mg Fiber: 5g

Creamy Avocado Zoodles

Creamy avocado sauce tossed with zucchini noodles, creating a light and satisfying keto vegan dinner.

Preparation Time: 10 minutes
Cooking Time: 5 minutes
Total Time: 15 minutes
Serving Size: 2

Ingredients:
2 medium zucchinis, spiralized
2 ripe avocados
2 tablespoons olive oil
2 cloves garlic, minced
Salt and pepper to taste

Directions:
1. In a blender or food processor, combine ripe avocados, olive oil, minced garlic, salt, and pepper. Blend until smooth and creamy.
2. In a large skillet, heat the avocado sauce over low heat.
3. Add the zucchini noodles to the skillet and toss until well-coated. Cook for 2-3 minutes, just until heated through.
4. Serve hot.

Nutritional Info (per serving): Calories: 370 Protein: 8g (17%) Carbohydrates: 20g (9%) Fat: 32g (78%) Sodium: 20mg Potassium: 1240mg Fiber: 14g

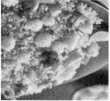

Cauliflower Rice Stir-Fry

A quick and flavorful stir-fry featuring cauliflower rice, tofu, and colorful vegetables, perfect for a satisfying keto vegan dinner.

Preparation Time: 15 minutes
Cooking Time: 10 minutes
Total Time: 25 minutes
Serving Size: 4

Ingredients:
1 medium head cauliflower, riced
1 block extra firm tofu, cubed
1 cup mixed vegetables (e.g. broccoli, bell peppers, and snap peas)
2 tablespoons coconut aminos (non-keto can use soy sauce)
2 tablespoons sesame oil

Directions:
1. In a large skillet or wok, heat sesame oil over medium heat. Add cubed tofu to skillet or wok and cook until golden brown on all sides.
2. Add mixed vegetables and sauté for 3-4 minutes until slightly tender.
3. Stir in cauliflower rice and cook for another 3 to 4 minutes.
4. Drizzle coconut aminos (or soy sauce) over the mixture. Toss to combine.
5. Serve hot.

Nutritional Info (per serving): Calories: 240 Protein: 15g (20%) Carbohydrates: 12g (7%) Fat: 15g (56%) Sodium: 250mg Potassium: 620mg Fiber: 5g

Vegan Creamed Spinach with Tofu

This creamy and satisfying dish combines nutrient-rich spinach with tofu for a protein-packed keto vegan dinner.

Preparation Time: 10 minutes
Cooking Time: 15 minutes
Total Time: 25 minutes
Serving Size: 4

Ingredients:

1 lb fresh spinach
1 block extra firm tofu, crumbled
1 cup coconut cream (from a can, make sure it's unsweetened and full-fat)
2 cloves garlic, minced
2 tablespoons coconut oil

Directions:

1. In a large skillet, heat coconut oil over medium heat. Add minced garlic and sauté for 1-2 minutes until fragrant.
2. Add fresh spinach to the skillet and cook until wilted.
3. Stir in crumbled tofu and coconut cream. Cook for an additional 5-7 minutes until heated through.
4. Serve hot.

Nutritional Info (per serving): Calories: 320 Protein: 16g (20%) Carbohydrates: 6g (7%) Fat: 28g (70%) Sodium: 180mg Potassium: 1220mg Fiber: 4g

Spaghetti Squash with Pesto and Cherry Tomatoes

This dish features roasted spaghetti squash topped with a vibrant basil pesto and fresh cherry tomatoes for a light and flavorful keto vegan dinner.

Preparation Time: 15 minutes
Cooking Time: 40 minutes
Total Time: 55 minutes
Serving Size: 2

Ingredients:

1 medium spaghetti squash
1 cup fresh basil leaves
1/2 cup pine nuts
2 tablespoons olive oil
1 cup cherry tomatoes, halved

Directions:

1. Preheat the oven to 375°F (190°C).

2. Cut the spaghetti squash in half lengthwise and scoop out the seeds. let the halves face side down on a baking sheet. Bake for about 40 minutes, or until the flesh is easily pierced with a fork.

3. While the squash is roasting, prepare the pesto. In a food processor, combine basil leaves, pine nuts, garlic, and olive oil. Blend until smooth. Season with salt to taste.

4. Once the squash is cooked, use a fork to scrape out the strands.

5. Toss the spaghetti squash with the pesto until well-coated.

6. Add cherry tomatoes and gently mix.

7. Serve warm.

(20%) Carbohydrates: 20g (7%) Fat: 30g (75%) Sodium: 150mg Potassium: 740mg Fiber: 6g Nutritional Info (per serving): Calories: 360 Protein: 10g

Vegan Cauliflower Alfredo with Spinach

Creamy cauliflower alfredo sauce served over sautéed spinach for a nutritious and satisfying keto vegan dinner.

Preparation Time: 10 minutes
Cooking Time: 20 minutes
Total Time: 30 minutes
Serving Size: 4
Ingredients:
1 medium head cauliflower, chopped
4 cups fresh spinach leaves
1/4 cup nutritional yeast
2 tablespoons olive oil
Salt and pepper to taste

Directions:

1. Steam or boil the cauliflower until tender. Drain and transfer to a blender.

2. Add nutritional yeast, salt, and pepper to the cauliflower in the blender. Blend until smooth and creamy.

3. In a large skillet, heat olive oil over medium heat. Add the spinach leaves and sauté for a minute or until wilted.

4. Serve the cauliflower alfredo sauce over the sautéed spinach.

Nutritional Info (per serving): Calories: 160 Protein: 8g (20%) Carbohydrates: 10g (6%) Fat: 11g (60%) Sodium: 120mg Potassium: 740mg Fiber: 5g

Stuffed Bell Peppers with Quinoa

These stuffed bell peppers are filled with a delicious mixture of quinoa, black beans, tomatoes, and spices, making for a satisfying and nutritious keto vegan dinner.

Preparation Time: 15 minutes

Cooking Time: 35 minutes
Total Time: 50 minutes
Serving Size: 4
Ingredients:
4 large bell peppers, tops removed and seeds removed
1 cup cooked quinoa
1 can (15 oz.) black beans, drained and rinsed
1 can (15 oz.) diced tomatoes
1 tablespoon olive oil
Directions:
1. Preheat the oven to 375°F (190°C).
2. In a large mixing bowl, combine cooked quinoa, black beans, and diced tomatoes.
3. Stuff each bell pepper with the quinoa mixture and place them in a baking dish.
4. Drizzle olive oil over the tops of the stuffed peppers.
5. Cover the baking dish with foil and bake for about 30-35 minutes, or until the peppers are tender.
6. Serve hot.
Nutritional Info (per serving): Calories: 290 Protein: 11g (16%) Carbohydrates: 47g (13%) Fat: 6g (18%) Sodium: 570mg Potassium: 1160mg Fiber: 14g

Vegan Zucchini Noodle Stir-Fry

This quick and flavorful stir-fry features zucchini noodles, tofu, and a savory sauce, providing a light yet satisfying keto vegan dinner option.
Preparation Time: 15 minutes
Cooking Time: 10 minutes
Total Time: 25 minutes
Serving Size: 2
Ingredients:
2 medium zucchinis, spiralized
1 block extra firm tofu, cubed
1/4 cup coconut aminos (or soy sauce for non-keto)
2 tablespoons sesame oil
2 cloves garlic, minced
Directions:
1. In a large skillet, heat sesame oil over medium heat. Add cubed tofu to the skillet and cook until golden brown on all sides.
2. Add minced garlic and sauté for 1-2 minutes until fragrant.
3. Add zucchini noodles to the skillet and drizzle with coconut aminos. Toss until well-coated and cook for 2-3 minutes, just until heated through.
4. Serve hot.
Nutritional Info (per serving): Calories: 360 Protein: 25g (20%) Carbohydrates: 12g (7%) Fat: 22g (56%) Sodium: 420mg Potassium: 960mg Fiber: 3g

Vegan Pesto Zoodles

This dish features spiralized zucchini noodles tossed in a vibrant basil pesto, creating a fresh and flavorful keto vegan dinner.

Preparation Time: 10 minutes
Cooking Time: 0 minutes
Total Time: 10 minutes
Serving Size: 2
Ingredients:
2 medium zucchinis, spiralized
1 cup fresh basil leaves
1/4 cup pine nuts
2 tablespoons olive oil
1/4 cup nutritional yeast (optional, for a cheesy flavor)
Directions:
1. In a food processor, combine fresh basil leaves, pine nuts, olive oil, and nutritional yeast (if using). Blend until smooth.
2. In a large bowl, toss the spiralized zucchini with the pesto sauce.
3. Serve chilled.
Nutritional Info (per serving): Calories: 280 Protein: 10g (14%) Carbohydrates: 10g (7%) Fat: 24g (77%) Sodium: 10mg Potassium: 840mg Fiber: 4g

Vegan Cauliflower Fried Rice

This low-carb alternative to traditional fried rice uses cauliflower rice and a medley of vegetables for a satisfying keto vegan dinner.

Preparation Time: 20 minutes
Cooking Time: 10 minutes
Total Time: 30 minutes
Serving Size: 4
Ingredients:
1 medium head cauliflower, riced
1 cup mixed vegetables (e.g., peas, carrots, bell peppers), diced
1/2 cup scallions, chopped
3 tablespoons coconut aminos (or soy sauce for non-keto)
2 tablespoons sesame oil
Directions:
1. In a large skillet or wok, heat sesame oil over medium heat. Add diced mixed vegetables and sauté for 3-4 minutes until slightly tender.
2. Stir in cauliflower rice and cook for an additional 3-4 minutes.
3. Drizzle coconut aminos (or soy sauce) over the mixture. Toss to combine.

4. Garnish with chopped scallions and serve hot.
Nutritional Info (per serving): Calories: 180 Protein: 5g (16%) Carbohydrates: 12g (7%) Fat: 14g (70%) Sodium: 480mg Potassium: 440mg Fiber: 4g

Dessert Recipes

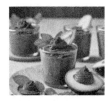

Chocolate Avocado Mousse

Creamy and rich, this chocolate avocado mousse is a decadent treat that's also packed with healthy fats.
Preparation Time: 10 minutes
Cooking Time: 0 minutes
Total Time: 10 minutes
Serving Size: 2
Ingredients:
2 ripe avocados
1/4 cup unsweetened cocoa powder
1/4 cup coconut milk
2-3 tablespoons low-carb sweetener (like erythritol or stevia), adjust to taste
1 teaspoon vanilla extract
Directions:
1. Cut avocados in half, remove the pit, and scoop out the flesh into a blender or food processor.
2. Add cocoa powder, coconut milk, sweetener, and vanilla extract.
3. Blend until smooth and creamy.
4. Divide into two serving glass cups and refrigerate for at least 2 hours before serving.
Nutritional Info (per serving): Calories: 230 Protein: 3g Carbohydrates: 12g Fat: 21g Sodium: 10mg Potassium: 585mg Fiber: 8g

Almond Butter Fat Bombs

These almond butter fat bombs are a quick, satisfying snack loaded with healthy fats.
Preparation Time: 10 minutes
Cooking Time: 0 minutes
Total Time: 10 minutes
Serving Size: 1 fat bomb
Ingredients:
1/2 cup almond butter
1/4 cup coconut oil, melted

2 tablespoons powdered erythritol (use any low-carb sweetener of choice)
1/2 teaspoon vanilla extract
Pinch of salt
Directions:
1. In a bowl, mix almond butter, melted coconut oil, erythritol, vanilla extract, and a pinch of salt until well combined.
2. Spoon the mixture into silicone molds or form into small balls and place on a parchment-lined tray.
3. Freeze for 30 minutes or until firm. Store in the refrigerator.
Nutritional Info (per serving): Calories: 90 Protein: 2g Carbohydrates: 2g Fat: 9g Sodium: 30mg Potassium: 45mg Fiber: 1g

Coconut Chia Pudding

Creamy coconut chia pudding is a simple and nutritious dessert option.
Preparation Time: 5 minutes
Cooking Time: 0 minutes
Total Time: 5 minutes
Serving Size: 1/2 cup
Ingredients:
1/4 cup chia seeds
1 cup coconut milk (full fat)
1 tablespoon low-carb sweetener (like erythritol or stevia), adjust to taste
1/2 teaspoon vanilla extract
Unsweetened coconut flakes for topping (optional)
Directions:
1. In a bowl, whisk together chia seeds, coconut milk, sweetener, and vanilla extract.
2. Let it sit for 15 minutes, stirring occasionally, until it thickens.
3. Put in the fridge for at least 2 hours or overnight.
4. Top with coconut flakes before serving, if desired.
Nutritional Info (per serving): Calories: 180 Protein: 4g Carbohydrates: 9g Fat: 14g Sodium: 10mg Potassium: 130mg Fiber: 7g

Lemon Coconut Fat Bombs

These tangy lemon coconut fat bombs are a refreshing treat that's both keto and vegan.
Preparation Time: 10 minutes
Cooking Time: 0 minutes
Total Time: 10 minutes
Serving Size: 1 fat bomb
Ingredients:
1/2 cup coconut butter

Zest of 1 lemon
2 tablespoons lemon juice
2 tablespoons powdered erythritol (use any low-carb sweetener of choice)
Unsweetened shredded coconut for rolling (optional)

Directions:

1. In a microwave-safe bowl, melt the coconut butter in short intervals until smooth.
2. Stir in the lemon zest, lemon juice, and sweetener until well combined.
3. Spoon the mixture into silicone molds or form into small balls and place on a parchment-lined tray.
4. Optional: Roll the fat bombs in shredded coconut.
5. Freeze for 30 minutes or until firm. Store in the refrigerator.

Nutritional Info (per serving): Calories: 90 Protein: 1g Carbohydrates: 2g Fat: 9g Sodium: 0mg Potassium: 10mg Fiber: 1g

Vanilla Almond Panna Cotta

This creamy vanilla almond panna cotta is a smooth and elegant dessert option.
Preparation Time: 10 minutes
Cooking Time: 10 minutes
Total Time: 4 hours (including chilling time)
Serving Size: 1/2 cup

Ingredients:
1 can (13.5 oz) full-fat coconut milk
1/4 cup almond butter
2 tablespoons powdered erythritol (use any low-carb sweetener of choice)
1 teaspoon vanilla extract
1 packet (2 1/4 teaspoons) unflavored gelatin

Directions:

1. In a saucepan, whisk together coconut milk, almond butter, sweetener, and vanilla extract. Heat over low-medium until it begins to simmer.
2. Sprinkle gelatin over the mixture and whisk until dissolved.
3. Pour into molds or ramekins and refrigerate for at least 4 hours or until set.

Nutritional Info (per serving): Calories: 180 Protein: 4g Carbohydrates: 4g Fat: 16g Sodium: 15mg Potassium: 160mg Fiber: 1g

Raspberry Coconut Chia Jam

This raspberry coconut chia jam is a delightful spread that's perfect for desserts or breakfast.
Preparation Time: 5 minutes
Cooking Time: 10 minutes
Total Time: 15 minutes
Serving Size: 2 tablespoons

Ingredients:
1 cup raspberries (fresh or frozen)
2 tablespoons chia seeds
2 tablespoons low-carb sweetener (like erythritol or stevia), adjust to taste
2 tablespoons unsweetened shredded coconut

1 tablespoon water

Directions:

1. In a saucepan, combine raspberries, chia seeds, sweetener, shredded coconut, and water.

2. Cook over medium heat, stirring occasionally, until the raspberries break down and the mixture thickens (about 10 minutes).

3. Allow the jam to cool before transferring it to a jar. Store in the refrigerator.

Nutritional Info (per serving): Calories: 40 Protein: 1g Carbohydrates: 5g Fat: 2g Sodium: 0mg Potassium: 50mg Fiber: 3g

No-Bake Coconut Cookies

These no-bake coconut cookies are a quick and satisfying treat.

Preparation Time: 10 minutes

Cooking Time: 0 minutes

Total Time: 10 minutes

Serving Size: 1 cookie

Ingredients:

1/2 cup coconut flour

1/4 cup coconut oil, melted

2 tablespoons powdered erythritol (use any low-carb sweetener of choice)

2 tablespoons unsweetened shredded coconut

1/2 teaspoon vanilla extract

Directions:

1. In a bowl, combine coconut flour, melted coconut oil, sweetener, shredded coconut, and vanilla extract.

2. Form the mixture into small cookies and place them on a parchment-lined tray.

3. Refrigerate for 30 minutes or until firm.

Nutritional Info (per serving): Calories: 90 Protein: 1g Carbohydrates: 4g Fat: 8g Sodium: 0mg Potassium: 10mg Fiber: 3g

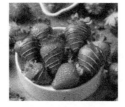

Chocolate Covered Strawberries

These chocolate-covered strawberries are a classic indulgence made keto and vegan.

Preparation Time: 10 minutes

Cooking Time: 5 minutes

Total Time: 15 minutes

Serving Size: 3 strawberries

Ingredients:

1 cup strawberries

2 tablespoons coconut oil

2 tablespoons unsweetened cocoa powder
2 tablespoons powdered erythritol (use any low-carb sweetener of choice)
A pinch of salt
Directions:
1. Rinse and pat dry the strawberries.
2. In a small saucepan, melt coconut oil over low heat. Stir in cocoa powder, sweetener, and a pinch of salt until smooth.
3. Dip each strawberry into the chocolate mixture, coating them evenly, and place them on a parchment-lined tray.
4. Refrigerate until the chocolate is set.
Nutritional Info (per serving): Calories: 70 Protein: 1g Carbohydrates: 5g Fat: 6g Sodium: 0mg Potassium: 120mg Fiber: 2g

Cinnamon Pecan Keto Fat Bombs

These cinnamon pecan fat bombs are a delightful blend of warm spices and crunchy pecans.
Preparation Time: 10 minutes
Cooking Time: 0 minutes
Total Time: 10 minutes
Serving Size: 1 fat bomb
Ingredients:
1/2 cup pecans, finely chopped
1/4 cup coconut oil, melted
2 tablespoons powdered erythritol (use any low-carb sweetener of choice)
1/2 teaspoon ground cinnamon
1/4 teaspoon vanilla extract
Directions:
1. In a bowl, combine chopped pecans, melted coconut oil, sweetener, ground cinnamon, and vanilla extract.
2. Spoon the mixture into silicone molds or form into small balls and place on a parchment-lined tray.
3. Freeze for 30 minutes or until firm. Store in the refrigerator.
Nutritional Info (per serving): Calories: 90 Protein: 1g Carbohydrates: 2g Fat: 9g Sodium: 0mg Potassium: 10mg Fiber: 1g

Matcha Chia Pudding

This matcha chia pudding is a vibrant and energizing dessert option.
Preparation Time: 5 minutes
Cooking Time: 0 minutes
Total Time: 5 minutes
Serving Size: 1/2 cup
Ingredients:
1/4 cup chia seeds
1 cup coconut milk (full fat)
2 teaspoons matcha powder
2 tablespoons low-carb sweetener (like erythritol or stevia), adjust to taste
1/2 teaspoon vanilla extract

Directions:

1. In a bowl, whisk together chia seeds, coconut milk, matcha powder, sweetener, and vanilla extract.
2. Let it sit for 15 minutes, stirring occasionally, until it thickens.
3. Put in the fridge for at least 2 hours or overnight.

Nutritional Info (per serving): Calories: 160 Protein: 3g Carbohydrates: 10g Fat: 11g Sodium: 10mg Potassium: 130mg Fiber: 7g

Brunch Recipes

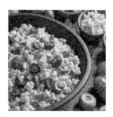

Avocado and Spinach Breakfast Bowl

This breakfast bowl is a nutritious and flavorful way to start your day.

Preparation Time: 10 minutes
Cooking Time: 5 minutes
Total Time: 15 minutes
Serving Size: 1 bowl

Ingredients:

1 avocado, sliced
1 cup fresh spinach leaves
2 tablespoons olive oil
1 tablespoon nutritional yeast
Salt and pepper to taste

Directions:

1. In a skillet, heat olive oil over medium heat. Add spinach and sauté until wilted.
2. Arrange the cooked spinach and sliced avocado in a bowl.
3. Sprinkle with nutritional yeast, salt, and pepper.
4. Serve warm.

Nutritional Info (per serving): Calories: 330 Protein: 6g (18%) Carbohydrates: 11g (7%) Fat: 30g (75%) Sodium: 15mg Potassium: 1200mg Fiber: 10g

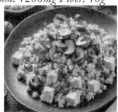

Tofu Scramble with Mushrooms

This tofu scramble is a satisfying and protein-packed brunch option.
Preparation Time: 10 minutes
Cooking Time: 10 minutes
Total Time: 20 minutes
Serving Size: 1 serving
Ingredients:
150g firm tofu, crumbled
1 cup mushrooms, sliced
2 tablespoons olive oil
1/2 teaspoon turmeric powder
Salt and pepper to taste
Directions:
1. In a skillet, heat olive oil over medium heat. Add mushrooms and sauté until golden.
2. Add crumbled tofu and turmeric powder. Cook for another 5 minutes, stirring occasionally.
3. Season with salt and pepper. Serve hot.
Nutritional Info (per serving): Calories: 250 Protein: 18g (28%) Carbohydrates: 6g (10%) Fat: 18g (65%) Sodium: 10mg Potassium: 420mg Fiber: 2g

Coconut Chia Pudding with Berries

This coconut chia pudding is a creamy, low-carb option topped with fresh berries.
Preparation Time: 5 minutes
Cooking Time: 0 minutes
Total Time: 5 minutes (plus chilling time)
Serving Size: 1 serving
Ingredients:
2 tablespoons chia seeds
1/2 cup coconut milk (full fat)
1/4 cup mixed berries (strawberries, blueberries, raspberries)
1 tablespoon unsweetened coconut flakes
1/2 teaspoon low-carb sweetener (like erythritol or stevia), optional
Directions:
1. In a bowl, combine chia seeds and coconut milk. Mix well and let it sit for 15 minutes, stirring occasionally.
2. Top with mixed berries, coconut flakes, and sweetener (if using).
3. Put in the fridge for at least 2to3 hours or overnight.
Nutritional Info (per serving): Calories: 230 Protein: 6g (10%) Carbohydrates: 14g (6%) Fat: 17g (70%) Sodium: 10mg Potassium: 210mg Fiber: 8g

Smashed Avocado and Tomato Toast

This smashed avocado toast is a quick and flavorful brunch option.
Preparation Time: 5 minutes
Cooking Time: 0 minutes

Total Time: 5 minutes
Serving Size: 1 serving
Ingredients:
1 slice of keto-friendly bread (e.g., almond flour bread)
1/2 avocado, mashed
1 small tomato, sliced
Salt and pepper to taste
Fresh basil leaves for garnish (optional)
Directions:
1. Toast the keto-friendly bread to your desired level of crispiness.
2. Spread mashed avocado onto the toast.
3. Top with tomato slices, salt, and pepper. You can garnish with fresh basil leaves if you want.
4. Serve immediately.
Nutritional Info (per serving): Calories: 220 Protein: 4g (18%) Carbohydrates: 10g (5%) Fat: 18g (77%) Sodium: 170mg Potassium: 660mg Fiber: 7g

Vegan Keto Pancakes

These vegan keto pancakes are fluffy and delicious, without the carbs.
Preparation Time: 10 minutes
Cooking Time: 10 minutes
Total Time: 20 minutes
Serving Size: 2 pancakes
Ingredients:
1/4 cup coconut flour
1/4 cup unsweetened almond milk
2 tablespoons ground flaxseed
1 tablespoon coconut oil (for cooking)
1/2 teaspoon baking powder
Directions:
1. In a bowl, mix coconut flour, almond milk, ground flaxseed, and baking powder until well combined.
2. Heat the oil in a skillet or saucepan over medium heat.
3. Pour the batter into the skillet to form pancakes. Cook for 2to3 minutes on both side, or until golden brown.
4. Serve hot with your favorite toppings.
Nutritional Info (per serving): Calories: 220 Protein: 7g (18%) Carbohydrates: 11g (8%) Fat: 16g (70%) Sodium: 90mg Potassium: 170mg Fiber: 8g

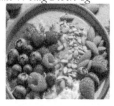

Almond Butter and Berry Smoothie Bowl

This smoothie bowl is a creamy, nutty delight topped with fresh berries.

Preparation Time: 5 minutes
Cooking Time: 0 minutes
Total Time: 5 minutes
Serving Size: 1 bowl

Ingredients:

2 tablespoons almond butter
1/2 cup unsweetened almond milk
1/4 cup mixed berries (strawberries, blueberries, raspberries)
1 tablespoon chia seeds
1 tablespoon sliced almonds

Directions:

1. In a blender, combine almond butter and almond milk. Blend until smooth.
2. Pour into a bowl and top with mixed berries, chia seeds, and sliced almonds.
3. Serve immediately.

Nutritional Info (per serving): Calories: 350 Protein: 10g (20%) Carbohydrates: 15g (8%) Fat: 28g (69%) Sodium: 110mg Potassium: 330mg Fiber: 9g

Vegan Keto Breakfast Burrito

This breakfast burrito is a hearty, satisfying option for brunch.
Preparation Time: 10 minutes
Cooking Time: 10 minutes
Total Time: 20 minutes
Serving Size: 1 burrito
Ingredients:
2 large collard green leaves
1/4 cup firm tofu, crumbled
2 tablespoons avocado, sliced
1 tablespoon nutritional yeast
1 tablespoon olive oil
Directions:
1. In a skillet or saucepan, heat olive oil over medium heat. Add crumbled tofu and sauté until golden brown.
2. Steam collard green leaves for 2 minutes to soften.
3. Lay out the collard green leaves and fill with tofu, avocado, and nutritional yeast.
4. Fold like a burrito and serve.
Nutritional Info (per serving): Calories: 290 Protein: 17g (23%) Carbohydrates: 11g (7%) Fat: 20g (62%) Sodium: 150mg Potassium: 670mg Fiber: 7g

Chia Seed Pudding with Almond Butter

This chia seed pudding is a creamy, nutty delight perfect for brunch.
Preparation Time: 5 minutes
Cooking Time: 0 minutes
Total Time: 5 minutes (plus chilling time)
Serving Size: 1 serving
Ingredients:
2 tablespoons chia seeds
1/2 cup unsweetened almond milk
1 tablespoon almond butter
1/2 teaspoon low-carb sweetener (like erythritol or stevia), optional
Sliced strawberries for garnish
Directions:
1. In a bowl, combine chia seeds, almond milk, almond butter, and sweetener (if using). Mix well.
2. Put in the fridge for at least 2 hours or overnight.
3. Top with sliced strawberries before serving.
Nutritional Info (per serving): Calories: 210 Protein: 8g (16%) Carbohydrates: 12g (8%) Fat: 15g (65%) Sodium: 70mg Potassium: 280mg Fiber: 9g

Vegan Keto Breakfast Tacos
These breakfast tacos are a savory and flavorful option for a satisfying brunch.
Preparation Time: 10 minutes
Cooking Time: 10 minutes
Total Time: 20 minutes
Serving Size: 2 tacos
Ingredients:
4 small keto-friendly tortillas (e.g., almond flour tortillas)
1/4 cup black beans, cooked
2 tablespoons salsa
1/4 avocado, sliced
2 tablespoons fresh cilantro, chopped
Directions:
1. Warm the tortillas in a dry skillet over medium heat for about 20 seconds on each side.
2. Fill each tortilla with black beans, salsa, avocado slices, and cilantro.
3. Fold the tortillas in half and serve.
Nutritional Info (per serving): Calories: 220 Protein: 6g (11%) Carbohydrates: 14g (8%) Fat: 16g (65%) Sodium: 160mg Potassium: 310mg Fiber: 9g

Vegan Keto Breakfast Salad
This breakfast salad is a fresh and satisfying way to start your day.
Preparation Time: 15 minutes
Cooking Time: 0 minutes
Total Time: 15 minutes
Serving Size: 1 salad
Ingredients:
2 cups mixed salad greens
1/4 cup cherry tomatoes, halved
1/4 avocado, sliced
2 tablespoons pumpkin seeds
2 tablespoons olive oil
Directions:
1. Arrange mixed greens, cherry tomatoes, avocado slices, and pumpkin seeds on a plate.
2. Drizzle olive oil over the salad.
3. Toss gently and serve.
Nutritional Info (per serving): Calories: 280 Protein: 5g (7%) Carbohydrates: 8g (6%) Fat: 26g (79%) Sodium: 20mg Potassium: 450mg Fiber: 6g

Drink Recipes

Green Keto Smoothie

This green keto smoothie is packed with nutrients and perfect for a quick breakfast.
Preparation Time: 5 minutes
Cooking Time: 0 minutes
Total Time: 5 minutes
Serving Size: 1 smoothie
Ingredients:
1 cup unsweetened almond milk
1/2 avocado
1 cup spinach leaves
1 tablespoon chia seeds
1 teaspoon low-carb sweetener (like erythritol or stevia), optional
Directions:
1. Combine almond milk, avocado, spinach, and chia seeds in a blender.
2. Blend until smooth.
3. Taste and add sweetener if desired.
4. Pour into a glass and serve.
Nutritional Info (per serving): Calories: 220 Protein: 5g (9%) Carbohydrates: 11g (7%) Fat: 18g (74%) Sodium: 160mg Potassium: 620mg Fiber: 9g

Iced Matcha Latte

This iced matcha latte is a refreshing and energizing drink.
Preparation Time: 5 minutes
Cooking Time: 0 minutes
Total Time: 5 minutes
Serving Size: 1 latte
Ingredients:
1 teaspoon matcha powder
1 cup unsweetened almond milk
1 tablespoon coconut cream
1/2 teaspoon low-carb sweetener (like erythritol or stevia), optional
Ice cubes
Directions:

1. In a glass, whisk matcha powder with a little hot water to form a paste.
2. Add almond milk, coconut cream, and sweetener (if using). Stir well.
3. Add ice cubes and stir until cold.

Nutritional Info (per serving): Calories: 60 Protein: 1g (7%) Carbohydrates: 3g (5%) Fat: 5g (70%) Sodium: 180mg Potassium: 40mg Fiber: 1g

Turmeric Golden Milk

This turmeric golden milk is a soothing and anti-inflammatory drink.

Preparation Time: 5 minutes
Cooking Time: 5 minutes
Total Time: 10 minutes
Serving Size: 1 cup

Ingredients:
1 cup unsweetened coconut milk
1/2 teaspoon ground turmeric
1/4 teaspoon ground cinnamon
A pinch of black pepper (enhances absorption of turmeric)
1 teaspoon low-carb sweetener (like erythritol or stevia), optional

Directions:
1. in a small saucepan, whisk together coconut milk, turmeric, cinnamon, black pepper, and sweetener (if using).
2. Heat over low-medium heat until warm, but not boiling.
3. Pour into a cup and enjoy.

Nutritional Info (per serving): Calories: 60 Protein: 1g (7%) Carbohydrates: 2g (3%) Fat: 5g (70%) Sodium: 40mg Potassium: 60mg Fiber: 1g

Cucumber Mint Lemonade

This cucumber mint lemonade is a refreshing and hydrating drink.
Preparation Time: 10 minutes
Cooking Time: 0 minutes
Total Time: 10 minutes
Serving Size: 1 glass
Ingredients:
1/2 cucumber, sliced
A handful of fresh mint leaves
Juice of 1 lemon
1 tablespoon low-carb sweetener (stevia or erythritol), optional
Water
Directions:
1. In a blender, combine cucumber, mint leaves, lemon juice, sweetener (if using), and a splash of water.
2. Blend until smooth and then Strain to remove any pulp.
4. Add water to achieve desired consistency and taste. Stir well. Enjoy!
Nutritional Info (per serving): Calories: 20 Protein: 0g Carbohydrates: 5g (10%) Fat: 0g Sodium: 0mg Potassium: 90mg Fiber: 1g

Berry Chia Fresca

This berry chia fresca is a hydrating and fiber-rich drink.
Preparation Time: 5 minutes
Cooking Time: 0 minutes
Total Time: 5 minutes
Serving Size: 1 glass
Ingredients:
1/4 cup mixed berries (strawberries, blueberries, raspberries)
1 tablespoon chia seeds
Juice of 1/2 lemon
1 teaspoon low-carb sweetener (like erythritol or stevia), optional
Water
Directions:
1. In a glass, combine mixed berries, chia seeds, lemon juice, and sweetener (if using).
2. Mash the berries slightly with a fork.
3. Add water and stir well.
4. Let it sit for a few minutes to allow chia seeds to expand. Enjoy!
Nutritional Info (per serving): Calories: 30 Protein: 1g (15%) Carbohydrates: 5g (8%) Fat: 1g (70%) Sodium: 0mg Potassium: 60mg Fiber: 3g

Ginger Lemon Turmeric Tea

This tea is a warming and immune-boosting elixir.
Preparation Time: 5 minutes
Cooking Time: 5 minutes

Total Time: 10 minutes
Serving Size: 1 cup
Ingredients:
1-inch piece of ginger, sliced
Juice of 1/2 lemon
1/2 teaspoon ground turmeric
A pinch of black pepper
1 teaspoon low-carb sweetener (like erythritol or stevia), optional
Directions:
1. In a small saucepan, combine ginger, lemon juice, turmeric, black pepper, and sweetener (if using) with 1 cup of water.
2. Simmer over low heat for 5 minutes.
3. Strain and pour into a cup.
Nutritional Info (per serving): Calories: 20 Protein: 0g Carbohydrates: 5g (10%) Fat: 0g Sodium: 0mg Potassium: 30mg Fiber: 1g

Coconut Almond Shake

This coconut almond shake is a creamy and satisfying treat.
Preparation Time: 5 minutes
Cooking Time: 0 minutes
Total Time: 5 minutes
Serving Size: 1 shake
Ingredients:
1/2 cup unsweetened almond milk
2 tablespoons coconut cream
1 tablespoon almond butter
1 teaspoon low-carb sweetener (like erythritol or stevia), optional
Ice cubes
Directions:
1. In a blender, combine almond milk, coconut cream, almond butter, and sweetener (if using).
2. Blend until smooth.
3. Add ice cubes and blend until well incorporated.
Nutritional Info (per serving): Calories: 160 Protein: 3g (8%) Carbohydrates: 5g (6%) Fat: 14g (76%) Sodium: 120mg Potassium: 110mg Fiber: 2g

Spicy Jalapeño Limeade

This spicy jalapeño limeade is a zesty and invigorating drink.
Preparation Time: 10 minutes

Cooking Time: 5 minutes
Total Time: 15 minutes
Serving Size: 1 glass
Ingredients:
Juice of 2 limes
1 small jalapeño pepper, sliced
1 teaspoon low-carb sweetener (like erythritol or stevia), optional
Water
Ice cubes
Directions:
1. In a small saucepan, combine lime juice, jalapeño slices, sweetener (if using), and 1 cup of water.
2. Bring to a gentle simmer and let it cook for 5 minutes.
3. Remove the saucepan from the heat and let it cool.
4. Strain and pour into a glass filled with ice cubes.
5. Top up with more water and stir well.
Nutritional Info (per serving): Calories: 15 Protein: 0g Carbohydrates: 4g (10%) Fat: 0g Sodium: 0mg Potassium: 30mg Fiber: 1g

Chocolate Avocado Smoothie

This chocolate avocado smoothie is a rich and creamy indulgence.
Preparation Time: 5 minutes
Cooking Time: 0 minutes
Total Time: 5 minutes
Serving Size: 1 smoothie
Ingredients:
1/2 avocado
2 tablespoons unsweetened cocoa powder
1 tablespoon low-carb sweetener of choice (erythritol or stevia), optional
1 cup unsweetened almond milk
Ice cubes
Directions:
1. In a blender, combine avocado, cocoa powder, sweetener (if using), almond milk, and ice cubes.
2. Blend until smooth.
Nutritional Info (per serving): Calories: 170 Protein: 4g (9%) Carbohydrates: 11g (6%) Fat: 14g (74%) Sodium: 170mg Potassium: 500mg Fiber: 7g

Raspberry Coconut Smoothie

This raspberry coconut smoothie is a fruity and refreshing delight.

Preparation Time: 5 minutes
Cooking Time: 0 minutes
Total Time: 5 minutes
Serving Size: 1 smoothie
Ingredients:
1/2 cup frozen raspberries
2 tablespoons coconut cream
1 tablespoon chia seeds
1 teaspoon low-carb sweetener (like erythritol or stevia), optional
1 cup unsweetened almond milk
Directions:
1. In a blender, combine frozen raspberries, coconut cream, chia seeds, sweetener (if using), and almond milk.
2. Blend until smooth. Remove from the blender and serve
Nutritional Info (per serving): Calories: 140 Protein: 3g (9%) Carbohydrates: 10g (7%) Fat: 10g (64%) Sodium: 200mg Potassium: 150mg Fiber: 7g

Minty Cucumber Cooler

This minty cucumber cooler is a hydrating and invigorating drink.
Preparation Time: 10 minutes
Cooking Time: 0 minutes
Total Time: 10 minutes
Serving Size: 1 glass
Ingredients:
1/2 cucumber, sliced
A handful of fresh mint leaves
Juice of 1 lime
1 teaspoon low-carb sweetener (like erythritol or stevia), optional
Sparkling water
Directions:
1. In a glass, muddle cucumber slices and mint leaves.
2. Add lime juice and sweetener (if using). Stir well.
3. Fill the glass with sparkling water and stir gently.
Nutritional Info (per serving): Calories: 15 Protein: 0g Carbohydrates: 4g (10%) Fat: 0g Sodium: 0mg Potassium: 80mg Fiber: 1g

Blueberry Almond Shake

This blueberry almond shake is a creamy and antioxidant-rich beverage.
Preparation Time: 5 minutes
Cooking Time: 0 minutes
Total Time: 5 minutes
Serving Size: 1 shake
Ingredients:
1/4 cup frozen blueberries
2 tablespoons almond butter
1 tablespoon erythritol (or sweetener of chioc), optional

1 cup unsweetened almond milk
Ice cubes
Directions:
1. In a blender, combine frozen blueberries, almond butter, sweetener (if using), almond milk, and ice cubes.
2. Blend until smooth. Remove from the blender and serve immediately
Nutritional Info (per serving): Calories: 190Protein: 5g (10%) Carbohydrates: 9g (6%) Fat: 16g (76%) Sodium: 190mg Potassium: 170mg Fiber: 3g

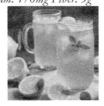

Lemon Ginger Kombucha

This lemon ginger kombucha is a probiotic-rich and digestive-aiding beverage.
Preparation Time: 5 minutes
Cooking Time: 0 minutes
Total Time: 5 minutes
Serving Size: 1 glass
Ingredients:
1 cup plain kombucha
Juice of 1/2 lemon
1-inch piece of ginger, grated
1 teaspoon low-carb sweetener (like erythritol or stevia), optional
Ice cubes
Directions:
1. In a glass, combine kombucha, lemon juice, grated ginger, and sweetener (if using). Stir well.
2. Add ice cubes and enjoy.
Nutritional Info (per serving): Calories: 15 Protein: 0g Carbohydrates: 3g (8%) Fat: 0g Sodium: 10mg Potassium: 20mg Fiber: 0g

Coconut Pineapple Smoothie

This coconut pineapple smoothie is a tropical and creamy treat.
Preparation Time: 5 minutes
Cooking Time: 0 minutes
Total Time: 5 minutes
Serving Size: 1 smoothie
Ingredients:
1/2 cup frozen pineapple chunks
2 tablespoons coconut cream
1 tablespoon chia seeds
1 teaspoon low-carb sweetener (like erythritol or stevia), optional

1 cup unsweetened almond milk

Directions:

1. In a blender, combine frozen pineapple chunks, coconut cream, chia seeds, sweetener (if using), and almond milk.

2. Blend until smooth. Remove from the blender and serve. Enjoy!

Nutritional Info (per serving): Calories: 180 Protein: 3g (7%) Carbohydrates: 15g (8%) Fat: 13g (65%) Sodium: 220mg Potassium: 190mg Fiber: 6g

Vanilla Almond Milk

This homemade vanilla almond milk is a creamy and versatile base for various drinks.

Preparation Time: 10 minutes

Cooking Time: 0 minutes

Total Time: 10 minutes

Serving Size: About 4 cups

Ingredients:

1 cup raw almonds, soaked overnight

4 cups water

1 teaspoon vanilla extract

1 teaspoon low-carb sweetener (like erythritol or stevia), optional

A pinch of salt

Directions:

1. Rinse soaked almonds and blend them with 4 cups of water in a high-speed blender until smooth.

2. Strain through a nut milk bag or fine-mesh strainer into a large bowl.

3. Pour the strained liquid back into the blender and add vanilla extract, sweetener (if using), and a pinch of salt. Blend again.

4. Transfer the almond milk to a container and refrigerate. Shake before use.

Nutritional Info (per serving, about 1 cup): Calories: 40 Protein: 1g (10%) Carbohydrates: 2g (5%) Fat: 3g (67%) Sodium: 20mg Potassium: 50mg Fiber: 1g

Soup and Stew Recipes

Mushroom and Spinach Stew

A hearty stew filled with earthy mushrooms and nutrient-rich spinach in a savory broth.
Preparation Time: 10 minutes
Cooking Time: 30 minutes
Total Time: 40 minutes
Serving Size: 2

Ingredients:
8 oz mushrooms, sliced
4 cups fresh spinach
1 small onion, diced
4 cloves garlic, minced
4 cups vegetable broth

Directions:
1. In a large pot, sauté the onion and garlic until fragrant and translucent.
2. Add the mushrooms and cook for 4 to 5 minutes or until they release their moisture and start to brown.
3. Pour in the vegetable broth and bring to a simmer. Let it cook for 15 minutes.
4. Add the spinach and cook for another 5 minutes until wilted.
5. Season to taste and serve.

Nutritional Info (per serving): Calories: 90 Protein: 6g (27%) Carbohydrate: 14g (18%) Fat: 1g (55%) Sodium: 800mg Potassium: 950mg Fiber: 4g

Cauliflower and Broccoli Stew

A creamy stew featuring cauliflower and broccoli for a satisfying keto-friendly meal.
Preparation Time: 15 minutes
Cooking Time: 25 minutes
Total Time: 40 minutes
Serving Size: 4

Ingredients:
1 small head cauliflower, chopped
2 cups broccoli florets
1 cup unsweetened almond milk
2 cloves garlic, minced
4 tbsp nutritional yeast

Directions:
1. Steam or boil the cauliflower and broccoli until tender. Drain and set aside.
2. In a blender, combine almond milk, garlic, and nutritional yeast. Blend until smooth.
3. In a large pot, combine the cooked vegetables and the creamy mixture. Simmer for 10 minutes.
4. Season to taste and serve.

Nutritional Info (per serving): Calories: 90 Protein: 7g (31%) Carbohydrate: 12g (14%) Fat: 2g (55%) Sodium: 200mg Potassium: 600mg Fiber: 6g

Spicy Coconut Chickpea Stew

A spicy and aromatic stew featuring creamy coconut milk and protein-rich chickpeas.
Preparation Time: 15 minutes
Cooking Time: 30 minutes
Total Time: 45 minutes
Serving Size: 4
Ingredients:
2 cans (15 oz. each) chickpeas, drained and rinsed
1 can (13.5 oz.) full-fat coconut milk
2 tbsp red curry paste
1 cup cherry tomatoes, halved
2 cups spinach
Directions:
1. In a large pot, combine chickpeas, coconut milk, and red curry paste. Simmer for 15 minutes.
2. Add cherry tomatoes and cook for another 10 minutes.
3. Stir in the spinach and cook for about a minute or until wilted.
4. Adjust spice level if needed and serve. Enjoy!
Nutritional Info (per serving): Calories: 420 Protein: 15g (14%) Carbohydrate: 55g (30%) Fat: 20g (56%) Sodium: 400mg Potassium: 800mg Fiber: 15g

Zucchini and Bell Pepper Stew

A colorful stew with zucchini and bell peppers cooked in a flavorful tomato base.
Preparation Time: 10 minutes
Cooking Time: 25 minutes
Total Time: 35 minutes
Serving Size: 3
Ingredients:
2 medium zucchinis, sliced
2 bell peppers (any color), chopped
1 can (14 oz) diced tomatoes
1 small onion, diced
2 cloves garlic, minced
Directions:
1. In a large pot, sauté the onion and garlic until fragrant and translucent.
2. Add the zucchinis and bell peppers.
3. Cook until slightly tender, about 5 minutes.
4. Pour in the diced tomatoes and let it simmer for 15 minutes.
5. Season to taste and serve.
Nutritional Info (per serving): Calories: 80 Protein: 3g (15%) Carbohydrate: 18g (25%) Fat: 0.5g (10%) Sodium: 350mg Potassium: 900mg Fiber: 6g

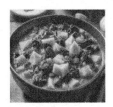

Artichoke and Spinach Stew

A creamy and rich stew featuring artichoke hearts and nutrient-packed spinach.
Preparation Time: 20 minutes
Cooking Time: 30 minutes
Total Time: 50 minutes
Serving Size: 4
Ingredients:
1 can (14 oz.) artichoke hearts, drained and chopped
4 cups fresh spinach
1 cup unsweetened almond milk
2 cloves garlic, minced
4 tbsp nutritional yeast
Directions:
1. In a blender, combine almond milk, garlic, and nutritional yeast. Blend until smooth.
2. In a large pot, add the artichoke hearts and creamy mixture. Simmer for 20 minutes.
3. Stir in the spinach and cook until wilted, for a minute or more.
4. Season to taste and serve.
Nutritional Info (per serving): Calories: 70 Protein: 6g (34%) Carbohydrate: 9g (21%) Fat: 2g (40%) Sodium: 250mg Potassium: 500mg Fiber: 4g

Cabbage and Seitan Stew

A hearty stew featuring cabbage and protein-packed seitan for a satisfying keto meal.
Preparation Time: 15 minutes
Cooking Time: 30 minutes
Total Time: 45 minutes
Serving Size: 3
Ingredients:
4 cups cabbage, chopped
8 oz seitan, sliced
1 small onion, diced
4 cups vegetable broth
2 tbsp olive oil
Directions:
1. In a large soup pot, heat the oil and sauté the onion until translucent, for about a minute.
2. Add the cabbage and seitan. Cook about 10 minutes or until cabbage is tender.
3. Pour in the vegetable broth and simmer for 20 minutes.

4. Season to taste and serve.

Nutritional Info (per serving): Calories: 240 Protein: 20g (33%) Carbohydrate: 15g (24%) Fat: 10g (37%) Sodium: 900mg Potassium: 600mg Fiber: 6g

Eggplant and Tomato Stew

A Mediterranean-inspired stew with eggplant and tomatoes for a burst of flavor.
Preparation Time: 20 minutes
Cooking Time: 25 minutes
Total Time: 45 minutes
Serving Size: 4
Ingredients:
1 large eggplant, cubed
1 can (14 oz) diced tomatoes
1 small onion, diced
2 cloves garlic, minced
2 tbsp olive oil
Directions:
1. In a large pot, heat the olive oil and sauté the onion and garlic until fragrant and translucent.
2. Add the eggplant and cook until slightly tender, about 10 minutes.
3. Pour in the diced tomatoes and let it simmer for 15 minutes.
4. Season to taste and serve.
Nutritional Info (per serving): Calories: 100 Protein: 3g (12%) Carbohydrate: 16g (25%) Fat: 4g (63%) Sodium: 250mg Potassium: 700mg Fiber: 8g

Lentil and Kale Stew

A protein-rich stew with lentils and nutrient-dense kale for a filling keto meal.
Preparation Time: 15 minutes
Cooking Time: 35 minutes
Total Time: 50 minutes
Serving Size: 4
Ingredients:
1 cup green lentils, rinsed
4 cups vegetable broth
2 cups kale, chopped
1 small onion, diced
2 cloves garlic, minced
Directions:

1. In a large pot, combine lentils, vegetable broth, onion, and garlic. Bring to a boil, then reduce heat and simmer for 30 minutes.
2. Add the kale and cook for another 5 minutes, until wilted.
3. Season to taste and serve.
Nutritional Info (per serving): Calories: 250 Protein: 18g (30%) Carbohydrate: 39g (39%) Fat: 1g (4%) Sodium: 900mg Potassium: 900mg Fiber: 16g

Asparagus and Almond Stew

A creamy and nutty stew featuring asparagus and almond butter for a unique flavor profile.
Preparation Time: 15 minutes
Cooking Time: 25 minutes
Total Time: 40 minutes
Serving Size: 3
Ingredients:
1 bunch asparagus, trimmed and chopped
2 tbsp almond butter
4 cups vegetable broth
2 cloves garlic, minced
2 tbsp olive oil
Directions:
1. In a large pot, heat the olive oil and sauté the garlic until fragrant.
2. Add the asparagus and cook until tender, about 10 minutes.
3. In a small bowl, whisk together almond butter and vegetable broth. Pour into the pot and simmer for 15 minutes.
4. Season to taste and serve.
Nutritional Info (per serving): Calories: 180 Protein: 8g (18%) Carbohydrate: 12g (27%) Fat: 14g (55%) Sodium: 750mg Potassium: 550mg Fiber: 6g

Tomato and Cucumber Stew

A refreshing stew with tomatoes and cucumbers, perfect for a light keto meal.
Preparation Time: 15 minutes
Cooking Time: 20 minutes
Total Time: 35 minutes
Serving Size: 2
Ingredients:
2 large tomatoes, chopped
2 cucumbers, chopped
1 small onion, diced
2 cloves garlic, minced
2 tbsp olive oil
Directions:
1. In a large pot, heat the olive oil and sauté the onion and garlic until fragrant.
Add the tomatoes and cook for 10 minutes until they break down.
Stir in the cucumbers and cook for another 5 minutes.
Season to taste and serve.

Nutritional Info (per serving): Calories: 180 Protein: 4g (9%) Carbohydrate: 24g (35%) Fat: 9g (45%) Sodium: 10mg Potassium: 1300mg Fiber

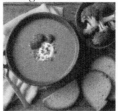

Creamy Broccoli Soup

This creamy broccoli soup is rich, comforting, and packed with nutrients.
Preparation Time: 10 minutes
Cooking Time: 20 minutes
Total Time: 30 minutes
Serving Size: 1 bowl
Ingredients:
2 cups broccoli florets
1 cup unsweetened almond milk
2 tablespoons olive oil
1/4 cup nutritional yeast
Salt and pepper to taste
Directions:
1. In a small cooking pot, heat olive oil over medium heat. Add broccoli florets and sauté for 5 minutes.
2. Add almond milk and bring to a simmer. Cook for 15 minutes or until broccoli is tender.
3. Transfer the mixture to a blender and add nutritional yeast, salt, and pepper. Blend until smooth.
4. Return the soup to the pot to reheat if necessary. Serve hot.
Nutritional Info (per serving): Calories: 250 Protein: 10g (16%) Carbohydrates: 12g (8%) Fat: 19g (69%) Sodium: 200mg Potassium: 800mg Fiber: 5g

Spicy Coconut Cauliflower Soup

This spicy coconut cauliflower soup is creamy, flavorful, and has a kick of heat.
Preparation Time: 10 minutes
Cooking Time: 25 minutes
Total Time: 35 minutes
Serving Size: 1 bowl
Ingredients:
2 cups cauliflower florets
1 can (14 oz) full-fat coconut milk
2 tablespoons coconut oil
1 teaspoon red pepper flakes (or to taste)
Salt to taste
Directions:

1. In a medium soup pot, heat coconut oil over medium heat. Add cauliflower and sauté for 5 minutes.
2. Pour in the coconut milk and red pepper flakes. Simmer until cauliflower is soft, for about 20 minutes.
3. Transfer the mixture to a blender or food processor and blend or process until smooth.
4. Return the soup to the pot to reheat if necessary. Add salt to taste. Serve hot.
Nutritional Info (per serving): Calories: 350 Protein: 5g (7%) Carbohydrates: 9g (6%) Fat: 35g (73%) Sodium: 60mg Potassium: 600mg Fiber: 3g

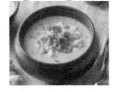

Zucchini and Basil Soup

This zucchini and basil soup is light, fresh, and bursting with herbaceous flavors.
Preparation Time: 10 minutes
Cooking Time: 20 minutes
Total Time: 30 minutes
Serving Size: 1 bowl
Ingredients:
2 medium zucchinis, chopped
1/4 cup fresh basil leaves
2 tablespoons olive oil
1/4 cup unsweetened almond milk
Salt and pepper to taste
Directions:
1. In a small cooking pot, heat olive oil over medium heat. Add chopped zucchinis and sauté for 5 minutes.
2. Add almond milk and basil leaves. Simmer for 15 minutes or until zucchinis are tender.
3. Transfer the mixture to a high powered blender and blend until smooth.
4. Return the soup to the pot to reheat if necessary. Add salt and pepper to taste. Serve hot.
Nutritional Info (per serving): Calories: 180 Protein: 5g (11%) Carbohydrates: 10g (7%) Fat: 14g (67%) Sodium: 30mg Potassium: 700mg Fiber: 3g

Cabbage and Turmeric Soup

This cabbage and turmeric soup is anti-inflammatory and packed with cruciferous goodness.
Preparation Time: 10 minutes
Cooking Time: 25 minutes
Total Time: 35 minutes
Serving Size: 1 bowl
Ingredients:
2 cups shredded cabbage
1 teaspoon ground turmeric
2 tablespoons olive oil
4 cups vegetable broth
Salt to taste
Directions:
1. In a small soup pot, heat olive oil over medium heat. Add shredded cabbage and sauté for 5 minutes.
2. Add ground turmeric and vegetable broth. Simmer for 20 minutes.
3. Add salt to taste. Serve hot.
Nutritional Info (per serving): Calories: 120 Protein: 2g (7%) Carbohydrates: 8g (6%) Fat: 9g (68%) Sodium: 800mg Potassium: 250mg Fiber: 3g

Spinach and Coconut Soup

This spinach and coconut soup is creamy, vibrant, and loaded with iron.
Preparation Time: 10 minutes
Cooking Time: 20 minutes
Total Time: 30 minutes
Serving Size: 1 bowl
Ingredients:
2 cups fresh spinach leaves
1 can (14 oz) full-fat coconut milk
2 tablespoons coconut oil
1/4 teaspoon ground nutmeg
Salt to taste
Directions:
1. In a small soup pot, heat the oil over medium heat. Add spinach and sauté for 3 minutes or until wilted.
2. Pour in the coconut milk and add ground nutmeg. Simmer for 15 minutes.
3. Transfer the mixture to a high powered blender and blend until smooth.
4. Return the soup to the pot to reheat if necessary. Add salt to taste. Serve hot.
Nutritional Info (per serving): Calories: 290 Protein: 3g (5%) Carbohydrates: 5g (6%) Fat: 29g (85%) Sodium: 20mg Potassium: 500mg Fiber: 2g

Avocado and Cucumber Soup

This avocado and cucumber soup is a refreshing, chilled option for warm days.
Preparation Time: 10 minutes

Cooking Time: 0 minutes
Total Time: 10 minutes
Serving Size: 1 bowl

Ingredients:
1 avocado
1/2 cucumber, peeled and chopped
1/4 cup fresh cilantro leaves
1 tablespoon lime juice
Salt to taste

Directions:
1. In a blender, combine avocado, cucumber, cilantro, lime juice, and a pinch of salt. Blend until smooth.
2. Taste and adjust salt if needed. Chill in the refrigerator before serving.

Nutritional Info (per serving): Calories: 250 Protein: 3g (5%) Carbohydrates: 14g (9%) Fat: 22g (80%) Sodium: 10mg Potassium: 760mg Fiber: 9g

Tomato and Basil Soup

This tomato and basil soup is a classic, bursting with tangy and herby flavors.
Preparation Time: 10 minutes
Cooking Time: 20 minutes
Total Time: 30 minutes
Serving Size: 1 bowl

Ingredients:
2 cups canned tomatoes
1/4 cup fresh basil leaves
2 tablespoons olive oil
2 cloves garlic, minced
Salt and pepper to taste

Directions:
1. In a small soup pot, heat olive oil over medium heat. Add minced garlic and sauté for 1 minute.
2. Add canned tomatoes (with juices) and basil leaves. Simmer for 15 minutes.
3. Use an immersion blender to blend the soup until smooth. Alternatively, transfer to a blender in batches.
4. Return the soup to the pot to reheat if necessary. Add salt and pepper to taste. Serve hot.

Nutritional Info (per serving): Calories: 190 Protein: 4g (8%) Carbohydrates: 10g (7%) Fat: 14g (63%) Sodium: 420mg Potassium: 780mg Fiber: 3g

Bell Pepper and Almond Soup

This bell pepper and almond soup is creamy, nutty, and vibrantly colored.
Preparation Time: 10 minutes
Cooking Time: 20 minutes
Total Time: 30 minutes
Serving Size: 1 bowl
Ingredients:
2 red bell peppers, roasted and peeled
1/4 cup almond butter
2 tablespoons olive oil
4 cups vegetable broth
Salt to taste
Directions:
1. In a small soup pot, heat olive oil over medium heat. Add roasted bell peppers and sauté for 5 minutes.
2. Add almond butter and vegetable broth. Simmer for 15 minutes.
3. Transfer the mixture to a high powered blender or food processor and blend or process until smooth.
4. Return the soup to the pot to reheat if necessary. Add salt to taste. Serve hot.
Nutritional Info (per serving): Calories: 280 Protein: 8g (12%) Carbohydrates: 10g (7%) Fat: 24g (77%) Sodium: 620mg Potassium: 600mg Fiber: 5g

Mushroom and Thyme Soup

This mushroom and thyme soup is earthy, aromatic, and perfect for mushroom lovers.
Preparation Time: 10 minutes
Cooking Time: 25 minutes
Total Time: 35 minutes
Serving Size: 1 bowl
Ingredients:
2 cups sliced mushrooms (any variety)
1/4 cup fresh thyme leaves
2 tablespoons olive oil
4 cups vegetable broth
Salt and pepper to taste
Directions:
1. In a small cooking pot, heat olive oil over medium heat. Add sliced mushrooms and thyme leaves. Sauté for 10 minutes.
2. Pour in the vegetable broth. Simmer for 15 minutes.
3. Add salt and pepper to taste. Serve hot.
Nutritional Info (per serving): Calories: 150 Protein: 5g (13%) Carbohydrates: 7g (5%) Fat: 11g (66%) Sodium: 620mg Potassium: 820mg Fiber: 3g

Spinach and Garlic Soup

This spinach and garlic soup is garlicky, nutrient-dense, and bursting with flavor.

Preparation Time: 10 minutes
Cooking Time: 15 minutes
Total Time: 25 minutes
Serving Size: 1 bowl
Ingredients:
2 cups fresh spinach leaves
4 cloves garlic, minced
2 tablespoons olive oil
4 cups vegetable broth
Salt to taste

Directions:
1. In a small cooking pot, heat olive oil over medium heat. Add minced garlic and sauté for 2 minutes or until fragrant.
2. Add fresh spinach leaves and sauté for another 3 minutes until wilted.
3. Pour in the vegetable broth. Simmer for 10 minutes.
4. Add salt to taste. Serve hot.

Nutritional Info (per serving): Calories: 140 Protein: 5g (13%) Carbohydrates: 7g (5%) Fat: 10g (64%) \ Sodium: 620mg Potassium: 870mg Fiber: 2g

Asparagus and Lemon Soup

This asparagus and lemon soup is bright, tangy, and celebrates the flavor of spring.
Preparation Time: 10 minutes
Cooking Time: 20 minutes
Total Time: 30 minutes
Serving Size: 1 bowl

Ingredients:
2 cups asparagus spears, chopped
Zest and juice of 1 lemon
2 tablespoons olive oil
4 cups vegetable broth
Salt and pepper to taste

Directions:
1. In a small cooking pot, heat olive oil over medium heat. Add chopped asparagus and sauté for 4 to 5 minutes.
2. Add vegetable broth and let it simmer. Cook for 15 minutes or until asparagus is tender.
3. Add lemon zest and juice. Stir well. Add salt and pepper to taste. Serve hot.

Nutritional Info (per serving): Calories: 160 Protein: 5g (13%) Carbohydrates: 8g (6%) Fat: 11g (63%) Sodium: 620mg Potassium: 770mg Fiber: 3g

Cauliflower and Rosemary Soup

This cauliflower and rosemary soup is fragrant, hearty, and perfect for a cozy evening.
Preparation Time: 10 minutes
Cooking Time: 25 minutes
Total Time: 35 minutes
Serving Size: 1 bowl
Ingredients:
2 cups cauliflower florets
2 teaspoons fresh rosemary, chopped
2 tablespoons olive oil
4 cups vegetable broth
Salt and pepper to taste
Directions:
1. In a small cooking pot, heat olive oil over medium heat. Add cauliflower florets to the heat pot with oil and sauté for 5 minutes.
2. Add vegetable broth to the pot and bring to a simmer. Cook for 20 minutes or until cauliflower is soft.
3. Stir in fresh rosemary. Add salt and pepper to taste. Serve hot.
Nutritional Info (per serving): Calories: 180 Protein: 4g (9%) Carbohydrates: 10g (7%) Fat: 14g (67%) Sodium: 620mg Potassium: 720mg Fiber: 4g

Appetizer Recipes

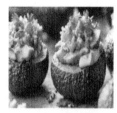

Avocado Stuffed Mushrooms

These delightful stuffed mushrooms are a perfect keto vegan appetizer, combining the creaminess of avocado with savory mushrooms.
Preparation Time: 15 minutes
Cooking Time: 15 minutes
Total Time: 30 minutes
Serving Size: 4 mushrooms per person
Ingredients:
16 large cremini mushrooms
2 ripe avocados
1/4 cup diced red bell pepper
2 cloves garlic, minced
2 tablespoons fresh lemon juice

Directions:
1. Preheat the oven to 375°F (190°C) and prepare a baking sheet.
2. Clean the mushrooms and remove the stems, creating a hollow space for the filling.
3. In a bowl, mash the avocados and mix in the diced red bell pepper, minced garlic, and lemon juice.
4. Stuff each mushroom cap with the avocado mixture and place them on the baking sheet.
5. Bake for 15 minutes or until the mushrooms are tender.
6. Serve hot and enjoy!

Nutritional Information (per serving): Calories: 120 Protein: 3g (10%) Carbohydrate: 7g (5%) Fat: 10g (75%) Sodium: 10mg Potassium: 430mg Fiber: 4g

Zucchini Fritters

These crispy zucchini fritters are a delightful keto vegan appetizer, perfect for snacking or as a side dish.

Preparation Time: 20 minutes
Cooking Time: 15 minutes
Total Time: 35 minutes
Serving Size: 2 fritters per person

Ingredients:
2 medium zucchinis, grated
1/4 cup almond flour
2 tablespoons ground flaxseed
2 cloves garlic, minced
2 tablespoons olive oil (for frying)

Directions:
1. Place the grated zucchini in a clean kitchen towel and squeeze out excess moisture.
2. In a large bowl, combine the zucchini, almond flour, ground flaxseed, and minced garlic. Mix until well combined.
3. Heat the olive oil in a skillet over medium heat.
4. Form small patties with the zucchini mixture and carefully place them in the hot skillet.
5. Cook for about 3-4 minutes on each side, or until golden brown and crispy.
6. Transfer the fritters to a plate lined with paper towels to remove excess oil.

Nutritional Information (per serving): Calories: 120 Protein: 4g (15%) Carbohydrate: 7g (5%) Fat: 9g (70%) Sodium: 5mg Potassium: 350mg Fiber: 3g

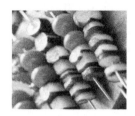

Cucumber and Tomato Skewers

These refreshing skewers combine the crispness of cucumber with the juiciness of cherry tomatoes for a light and flavorful keto vegan appetizer.

Preparation Time: 15 minutes
Cooking Time: 0 minutes
Total Time: 15 minutes
Serving Size: 2 skewers per person

Ingredients:
1 large cucumber, cut into chunks
1 cup cherry tomatoes
2 tablespoons olive oil
1 tablespoon fresh lemon juice
Salt and pepper to taste

Directions:
1. Thread cucumber chunks and cherry tomatoes onto skewers in an alternating pattern.
2. In a small bowl, whisk together the lemon juice, salt, olive oil and pepper.
3. Drizzle the dressing over the skewers and serve chilled.

Nutritional Information (per serving): Calories: 80 Protein: 1g (5%) Carbohydrate: 4g (10%) Fat: 7g (85%) Sodium: 5mg Potassium: 250mg Fiber: 1g

Stuffed Bell Peppers with cauliflower rice

These stuffed bell peppers are filled with a delicious mixture of cauliflower rice, black beans, and spices, creating a hearty keto vegan appetizer.

Preparation Time: 30 minutes
Cooking Time: 25 minutes
Total Time: 55 minutes
Serving Size: 1 stuffed pepper per person

Ingredients:
4 large bell peppers, any color
1 cup cauliflower rice
1/2 cup black beans, cooked and drained
1 teaspoon cumin
1 teaspoon paprika
Salt and pepper to taste

Directions:
1. Preheat the oven to 375°F (190°C).
2. Cut the tops off the bell peppers and remove the seeds and membranes.

3. In a large bowl, combine the cauliflower rice, black beans, cumin, paprika, salt, and pepper.
4. Stuff each bell pepper with the mixture and place them in a baking dish.
5. Cover with aluminum foil and bake for 25 minutes.
6. Remove the foil and bake for an additional 10 minutes, or until the peppers are tender.
7. Remove from the heath and enjoy!

Nutritional Information (per serving): Calories: 120 Protein: 5g (20%) Carbohydrate: 20g (10%) Fat: 1g (80%) Sodium: 15mg Potassium: 480mg Fiber: 7g

Cauliflower Buffalo Bites

These spicy cauliflower bites are a perfect keto vegan appetizer for those who crave the flavors of Buffalo wings without the meat.

Preparation Time: 15 minutes
Cooking Time: 25 minutes
Total Time: 40 minutes
Serving Size: 6 bites per person

Ingredients:
1 medium cauliflower head, cut into florets
1/2 cup almond flour
1/2 cup unsweetened almond milk
1/2 cup hot sauce
2 tablespoons olive oil

Directions:
1. Preheat the oven to 450°F (230°C).
2. In a bowl, whisk together almond flour and almond milk to create a batter.
3. Dip each cauliflower floret into the batter, allowing excess to drip off, and place on a baking sheet.
4. Bake until golden brown and crispy, for about 20-25 minutes.
5. In a separate bowl, combine hot sauce and olive oil.
6. Toss the baked cauliflower in the sauce mixture until well coated.

Nutritional Information (per serving): Calories: 150 Protein: 5g (15%) Carbohydrate: 8g (5%) Fat: 10g (80%) Sodium: 850mg Potassium: 440mg Fiber: 3g

Spinach and Artichoke Dip

This creamy spinach and artichoke dip is a classic keto vegan appetizer, perfect for dipping with low-carb crackers or vegetable sticks.

Preparation Time: 15 minutes
Cooking Time: 25 minutes
Total Time: 40 minutes
Serving Size: 2 tablespoons per person

Ingredients:
1 cup frozen spinach, thawed and drained
1 can (14 oz.) artichoke hearts, drained and chopped
1/2 cup unsweetened almond milk
1/4 cup nutritional yeast

2 cloves garlic, minced

Directions:

1. Preheat the oven to 375°F (190°C).

2. In a bowl, mix together the thawed spinach, chopped artichoke hearts, almond milk, nutritional yeast, and minced garlic.

3. Transfer the mixture to a baking dish and bake for 25 minutes, or until bubbly and lightly golden on top.

4. Serve warm with your choice of keto-friendly dippers.

Nutritional Information (per serving): Calories: 50 Protein: 4g (20%) Carbohydrate: 7g (10%) Fat: 2g (70%) Sodium: 200mg Potassium: 180mg Fiber: 4g

Coconut-Curry Cauliflower Bites

These flavorful cauliflower bites are coated in a coconut-curry sauce, creating a unique and delicious keto vegan appetizer.

Preparation Time: 15 minutes

Cooking Time: 30 minutes

Total Time: 45 minutes

Serving Size: 6 bites per person

Ingredients:

1 medium cauliflower head, cut into florets

1/2 cup coconut milk

2 tablespoons curry powder

2 tablespoons coconut oil

Salt and pepper to taste

Directions:

1. Preheat the oven to 450°F (230°C).

2. Place cauliflower florets on a baking sheet and drizzle with coconut oil. Season with salt and pepper.

3. Roast for 20-25 minutes, or until golden brown and crispy.

4. In a saucepan, combine coconut milk and curry powder. Heat over low heat, stirring until well combined.

5. Toss the roasted cauliflower in the coconut-curry sauce until evenly coated.

Nutritional Information (per serving): Calories: 150 Protein: 4g (15%) Carbohydrate: 8g (5%) Fat: 10g (80%) Sodium: 30mg Potassium: 430mg Fiber: 4g

Spicy Roasted Almonds

These spicy roasted almonds are a crunchy and flavorful keto vegan appetizer, perfect for snacking.

Preparation Time: 5 minutes

Cooking Time: 15 minutes

Total Time: 20 minutes

Serving Size: 1/4 cup per person

Ingredients:

2 cups raw almonds

1 tablespoon olive oil

1 teaspoon smoked paprika

1/2 teaspoon cayenne pepper (adjust to taste)

Salt to taste

Directions:

1. Preheat the oven to 350°F (175°C) and line a baking sheet with parchment paper.
2. In a bowl, toss the raw almonds with olive oil, smoked paprika, cayenne pepper, and salt until evenly coated.
3. Spread the almonds on the baking sheet in a single layer.
4. Roast for 10-15 minutes, stirring halfway through, until fragrant and golden.
5. Allow to cool before serving.

Nutritional Information (per serving): Calories: 160 Protein: 6g (15%) Carbohydrate: 6g (10%) Fat: 14g (75%) Sodium: 75mg Potassium: 210mg Fiber: 4g

Cabbage and Carrot Slaw

This refreshing slaw is a crunchy and tangy keto vegan appetizer that's quick to prepare.

Preparation Time: 10 minutes
Cooking Time: 0 minutes
Total Time: 10 minutes
Serving Size: 1/2 cup per person

Ingredients:

2 cups shredded cabbage
1 cup shredded carrots
2 tablespoons apple cider vinegar
1 tablespoon olive oil
1 teaspoon Dijon mustard

Directions:

1. In a large bowl, combine the carrots and shredded cabbage.
2. In a small bowl, whisk together the apple cider vinegar, olive oil, and dijon mustard.
3. Pour the dressing over the cabbage and carrots, tossing until well coated.
4. Allow the slaw to sit for a few minutes to let the flavors meld together before serving.

Nutritional Information (per serving): Calories: 70 Protein: 1g (5%) Carbohydrate: 6g (10%) Fat: 5g (75%) Sodium: 30mg Potassium: 160mg Fiber: 2g

Spicy Guacamole

This zesty guacamole is a classic keto vegan appetizer, perfect for dipping with low-carb tortilla chips or vegetable sticks.

Preparation Time: 10 minutes
Cooking Time: 0 minutes
Total Time: 10 minutes
Serving Size: 2 tablespoons per person

Ingredients:

2 ripe avocados
1/4 cup diced red onion
2 tablespoons fresh lime juice
1 jalapeño pepper, seeded and minced (or more to taste)

2 tablespoons chopped cilantro
Salt and pepper to taste
Directions:
1. Cut the avocados in half, remove the pit, and scoop the flesh into a medium mixing bowl.
2. Mash with a fork until desired consistency is reached.
3. Add the diced red onion, lime juice, minced jalapeño, chopped cilantro, salt, and pepper. Mix well.
4. Taste and adjust seasonings if necessary.
5. Serve immediately.
Nutritional Information (per serving): Calories: 80 Protein: 1g (5%) Carbohydrate: 5g (5%) Fat: 7g (70%) Sodium: 5mg Potassium: 250mg Fiber: 3g

Marinated Portobello Mushrooms

These marinated portobello mushrooms are a savory and satisfying keto vegan appetizer, perfect for grilling or baking.
Preparation Time: 20 minutes
Cooking Time: 15 minutes (grilling) or 25 minutes (baking)
Total Time: 35-45 minutes
Serving Size: 1 mushroom cap per person
Ingredients:
4 large portobello mushroom caps
1/4 cup balsamic vinegar
2 tablespoons olive oil
2 cloves garlic, minced
1 tablespoon fresh thyme leaves
Directions:
1. Clean the mushroom caps and remove the stems.
2. In a bowl, whisk together balsamic vinegar, olive oil, minced garlic, and fresh thyme leaves.
3. Place the mushroom caps in a shallow dish and pour the marinade over them. Let them marinate for at least 15 minutes or more.
4. Grill the mushrooms for about 7-8 minutes on each side, or bake at 375°F (190°C) for 25 minutes, until tender.
5. Serve hot.
Nutritional Information (per serving): Calories: 70 Protein: 2g (15%) Carbohydrate: 6g (10%) Fat: 5g (75%) Sodium: 10mg Potassium: 450mg Fiber: 1g

Cucumber Avocado Rolls

These cucumber avocado rolls are a light and refreshing keto vegan appetizer, perfect for a quick snack or appetizer.
Preparation Time: 15 minutes
Cooking Time: 0 minutes
Total Time: 15 minutes
Serving Size: 4 rolls per person
Ingredients:
2 large cucumbers
1 large avocado
1/4 cup sun-dried tomatoes, soaked and chopped
2 tablespoons fresh lemon juice
Fresh basil leaves, for garnish
Directions:
1. Cut the cucumbers lengthwise into thin strips using a vegetable peeler or a mandoline slicer.
2. In a bowl, mash the avocado and mix in the chopped sun-dried tomatoes and lemon juice.
3. Spread a thin layer of the avocado mixture onto each cucumber strip.
4. Roll up the cucumber strips and secure with a toothpick.
5. Garnish with fresh basil leaves and serve.
Nutritional Information (per serving): Calories: 90 Protein: 2g (10%) Carbohydrate: 7g (5%) Fat: 7g (85%) Sodium: 5mg Potassium: 380mg Fiber: 4g

Smoothies' Recipes

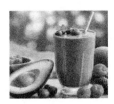

Berry Avocado Bliss Smoothie

This Berry Avocado Bliss Smoothie is a creamy and refreshing keto vegan drink packed with antioxidants and healthy fats.
Preparation Time: 5 minutes
Total Time: 5 minutes
Serving Size: 1 smoothie

Ingredients:
1/2 cup mixed berries (raspberries, blueberries, and strawberries)
1/4 avocado
1 tablespoon chia seeds
1 cup unsweetened almond milk
1 tablespoon coconut oil
Directions:
1. Add mixed berries, avocado, chia seeds, almond milk, and coconut oil to a blender.
2. Blend until smooth and creamy.
3. Pour into a glass and serve.
Nutritional Information (per serving): Calories: 250 Protein: 5g (20%) Carbohydrate: 10g (8%) Fat: 22g (78%) Sodium: 180mg Potassium: 380mg Fiber: 8g

Green Goddess Power Smoothie

The Green Goddess Power Smoothie is a nutrient-dense keto vegan delight, combining leafy greens with healthy fats for sustained energy.
Preparation Time: 7 minutes
Total Time: 7 minutes
Serving Size: 1 smoothie
Ingredients:
1 cup spinach leaves
1/4 avocado
1 tablespoon hemp seeds
1 cup unsweetened coconut milk
1 tablespoon almond butter
Directions:
1. Combine spinach leaves, avocado, hemp seeds, coconut milk, and almond butter in a blender.
2. Blend until smooth and creamy.
3. Pour into a glass and serve.
Nutritional Information (per serving): Calories: 280 Protein: 9g (15%) Carbohydrate: 8g (6%) Fat: 23g (78%) Sodium: 160mg Potassium: 530mg Fiber: 6g

Chocolate Almond Delight Smoothie

The Chocolate Almond Delight Smoothie is a decadent keto vegan treat, blending rich cacao with creamy almond butter for a delightful indulgence.
Preparation Time: 5 minutes
Total Time: 5 minutes
Serving Size: 1 smoothie

Ingredients:
1 tablespoon cacao powder
2 tablespoons almond butter
1/4 avocado
1 cup unsweetened almond milk
1 tablespoon chia seeds
Directions:
1. Add cacao powder, almond butter, avocado, almond milk, and chia seeds to a blender.
2. Blend until smooth and creamy.
3. Pour into a glass and serve.
Nutritional Information (per serving): Calories: 290 Protein: 8g (15%) Carbohydrate: 11g (7%) Fat: 25g (78%) Sodium: 180mg Potassium: 530mg Fiber: 8g

Coconut Berry Bliss Smoothie

The Coconut Berry Bliss Smoothie is a tropical keto vegan delight, combining the sweetness of berries with the creaminess of coconut.
Preparation Time: 5 minutes
Total Time: 5 minutes
Serving Size: 1 smoothie
Ingredients:
1/2 cup mixed berries (strawberries, blueberries and raspberries)
2 tablespoons shredded coconut
1/4 avocado
1 cup unsweetened coconut milk
1 tablespoon chia seeds
Directions:
1. Combine mixed berries, shredded coconut, avocado, coconut milk, and chia seeds in a blender.
2. Blend until smooth and creamy.
3. Pour into a glass and serve.
Nutritional Information (per serving): Calories: 280 Protein: 4g (15%) Carbohydrate: 11g (8%) Fat: 24g (77%) Sodium: 200mg Potassium: 380mg Fiber: 8g

Spinach and Almond Delight

This green smoothie is packed with nutrients and a subtle nutty flavor.
Preparation Time: 5 minutes
Total Time: 5 minutes
Serving Size: 1 smoothie
Ingredients:
2 cups fresh spinach leaves
2 tablespoons almond butter
1 cup unsweetened almond milk
1/4 teaspoon vanilla extract
1 tablespoon low-carb sweetener (like stevia or erythritol), optional
Directions:
1. Blend fresh spinach, almond butter, almond milk, vanilla extract, and sweetener (if using) until smooth.
2. Remove from the blender and serve chilled
Nutritional Info (per serving): Calories: 210 Protein: 8g (15%) Carbohydrates: 9g (5%) Fat: 17g (75%) Sodium: 280mg Potassium: 650mg Fiber: 5g

Coconut Berry Blast to continue from

This tropical-inspired smoothie is a burst of flavor with a creamy coconut twist.
Preparation Time: 5 minutes
Total Time: 5 minutes
Serving Size: 1 smoothie
Ingredients:
1/4 cup coconut cream
1/2 cup mixed berries (strawberries, blueberries, raspberries)
1 tablespoon chia seeds
1 cup unsweetened coconut milk
1 tablespoon erythritol (or low-carb sweetener of choice), optional
Directions:
1. Blend coconut cream, mixed berries, chia seeds, coconut milk, and sweetener (if using) until smooth.
Nutritional Info (per serving): Calories: 280 Protein: 4g (6%) Carbohydrates: 12g (7%) Fat: 24g (75%) Sodium: 40mg Potassium: 230mg Fiber: 8g

Vanilla Almond Joy

This smoothie brings together the classic combination of vanilla, almond, and coconut.
Preparation Time: 5 minutes
Total Time: 5 minutes
Serving Size: 1 smoothie
Ingredients:
1/2 teaspoon vanilla extract
2 tablespoons almond butter
1 tablespoon shredded unsweetened coconut
1 cup unsweetened almond milk

1 tablespoon erythritol (or low-carb sweetener of choice), optional

Directions:

1. Blend vanilla extract, almond butter, shredded coconut, almond milk, and sweetener (if using) until smooth.

Nutritional Info (per serving): Calories: 240 Protein: 7g (12%) Carbohydrates: 9g (5%) Fat: 20g (75%) Sodium: 220mg Potassium: 280mg Fiber: 5g

Cucumber Mint Cooler

This refreshing smoothie is perfect for a hot day with its cooling cucumber and invigorating mint.

Preparation Time: 5 minutes

Total Time: 5 minutes

Serving Size: 1 smoothie

Ingredients:

1/2 cucumber, sliced

A handful of fresh mint leaves

1 tablespoon lime juice

1 cup unsweetened almond milk

1 tablespoon erythritol (or low-carb sweetener of choice), optional

Directions:

1. Blend cucumber slices, fresh mint leaves, lime juice, almond milk, and sweetener (if using) until smooth.

Nutritional Info (per serving): Calories: 70 Protein: 2g (10%) Carbohydrates: 7g (4%) Fat: 4g (57%) Sodium: 200mg Potassium: 230mg Fiber: 2g

Chocolate Peanut Butter Powerhouse

Indulge in the decadent combination of chocolate and peanut butter with this protein-packed smoothie.

Preparation Time: 5 minutes

Total Time: 5 minutes

Serving Size: 1 smoothie

Ingredients:

2 tablespoons unsweetened cocoa powder

2 tablespoons peanut butter

1 cup unsweetened almond milk

1 tablespoon chia seeds

1 tablespoon stevia (or low-carb sweetener of choice), optional

Directions:

Blend cocoa powder, peanut butter, almond milk, chia seeds, and sweetener (if using) until smooth.

Nutritional Info (per serving): Calories: 280 Protein: 10g (18%) Carbohydrates: 12g (7%) Fat: 22g (73%) Sodium: 190mg Potassium: 350mg Fiber: 8g

Matcha Green Elixir

Boost your energy and focus with this vibrant matcha-infused smoothie.
Preparation Time: 5 minutes
Total Time: 5 minutes
Serving Size: 1 smoothie
Ingredients:
1 teaspoon matcha powder
1 tablespoon chia seeds
1 cup unsweetened almond milk
1 tablespoon stevia (or low-carb sweetener of choice), optional
A handful of baby spinach leaves
Directions:
1. Blend matcha powder, chia seeds, almond milk, sweetener (if using), and spinach until smooth.
Nutritional Info (per serving): Calories: 80 Protein: 3g (15%) Carbohydrates: 7g (4%) Fat: 5g (56%) Sodium: 250mg Potassium: 220mg Fiber: 4g

Turmeric Golden Glow

This anti-inflammatory smoothie gets its vibrant color and health benefits from turmeric.
Preparation Time: 5 minutes
Total Time: 5 minutes
Serving Size: 1 smoothie
Ingredients:
1 teaspoon ground turmeric
1/2 teaspoon ground ginger
1 tablespoon chia seeds
1 cup unsweetened almond milk
1 tablespoon stevia (or low-carb sweetener of choice), optional
Directions:
1. Blend ground turmeric, ground ginger, chia seeds, almond milk, and sweetener (if using) until smooth.
Nutritional Info (per serving): Calories: 60 Protein: 2g (13%) Carbohydrates: 7g (4%) Fat: 3g (45%) Sodium: 250mg Potassium: 220mg Fiber: 4g

Raspberry Coconut Refresher

This vibrant smoothie is a delightful combination of tart raspberries and creamy coconut.
Preparation Time: 5 minutes
Total Time: 5 minutes
Serving Size: 1 smoothie
Ingredients:
1/2 cup frozen raspberries
2 tablespoons coconut cream

1 cup unsweetened almond milk
1 tablespoon chia seeds
1 tablespoon stevia (or low-carb sweetener of choice), optional
Directions:
1. Blend frozen raspberries, coconut cream, almond milk, chia seeds, and sweetener (if using) until smooth.
Nutritional Info (per serving): Calories: 120 Protein: 2g (7%) Carbohydrates: 8g (6%) Fat: 9g (67%) Sodium: 160mg Potassium: 190mg Fiber: 6g

Pineapple Ginger Zing

This zesty smoothie combines tropical pineapple with the invigorating kick of ginger.
Preparation Time: 5 minutes
Total Time: 5 minutes
Serving Size: 1 smoothie
Ingredients:
1/2 cup frozen pineapple chunks
1-inch piece of ginger, grated
1 tablespoon chia seeds
1 cup unsweetened almond milk
1 tablespoon low-carb sweetener (like stevia or erythritol), optional
Directions:
1. Blend frozen pineapple chunks, grated ginger, chia seeds, almond milk, and sweetener (if using) until smooth.
Nutritional Info (per serving): Calories: 130 Protein: 2g (8%) Carbohydrates: 11g (6%) Fat: 9g (60%) Sodium: 160mg Potassium: 220mg Fiber: 5g

Chocolate Mint Marvel

This smoothie is like a refreshing mint chocolate chip dessert in a glass.
Preparation Time: 5 minutes
Total Time: 5 minutes
Serving Size: 1 smoothie
Ingredients:
2 tablespoons unsweetened cocoa powder
A handful of fresh mint leaves
1 cup unsweetened almond milk
1 tablespoon chia seeds
1 tablespoon low-carb sweetener (like erythritol, stevia or sweetener of choice), optional
Directions:
1. Blend cocoa powder, fresh mint leaves, almond milk, chia seeds, and sweetener (if using) until smooth.
Nutritional Info (per serving): Calories: 100 Protein: 3g (13%) Carbohydrates: 8g (5%) Fat: 7g (63%) Sodium: 180mg Potassium: 250mg Fiber: 6g

Lemon Blueberry Blast

This zesty smoothie combines the bright flavors of lemon with the sweetness of blueberries.
Preparation Time: 5 minutes
Total Time: 5 minutes
Serving Size: 1 smoothie

Ingredients:
Juice of 1 lemon
1/2 cup frozen blueberries
1 cup unsweetened almond milk
1 tablespoon chia seeds
1 tablespoon erythritol (or low-carb sweetener of choice), optional

Directions:
1. Blend lemon juice, frozen blueberries, almond milk, chia seeds, and sweetener (if using) until smooth.

Nutritional Info (per serving): Calories: 120 Protein: 3g (9%) Carbohydrates: 10g (7%) Fat: 8g (60%) Sodium: 160mg Potassium: 230mg Fiber: 5g

Dressing Recipes

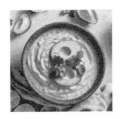

Creamy Avocado Lime Dressing

This creamy avocado lime dressing is a perfect addition to your keto vegan salads, adding richness and tanginess.
Preparation Time: 10 minutes
Total Time: 10 minutes
Serving Size: 2 tablespoons
Ingredients:
1 ripe avocado
Juice of 2 limes
2 tablespoons olive oil
Salt and pepper to taste
2 tablespoons water (adjust for desired consistency)
Directions:
1. Scoop out the flesh of the avocado and place it in a blender.
2. Add lime juice, olive oil, salt, pepper, and water.
3. Blend until smooth and creamy. Adjust water if needed for desired consistency.
4. Store dressing in an airtight container and keep in the fridge, use dressing within 5 days.
Nutritional Information (per serving): Calories: 90 Protein: 1g (20%) Carbohydrate: 3g (7%) Fat: 8g (73%) Sodium: 5mg Potassium: 260mg Fiber: 2g

Lemon Tahini Dressing

This zesty lemon tahini dressing adds a burst of flavor to your keto vegan salads, creating a creamy and tangy sensation.
Preparation Time: 5 minutes
Total Time: 5 minutes
Serving Size: 2 tablespoons
Ingredients:
2 tablespoons tahini
Juice of 1 lemon
2 tablespoons water
1 clove garlic, minced
Salt to taste
Directions:
1. In a small bowl, whisk together tahini, lemon juice, water, minced garlic, and salt until well combined.

2. Adjust water as needed for desired consistency.
3. Transfer dressing into an airtight container and store in the fridge, use dressing within 5 days.
Nutritional Information (per serving): Calories: 60 Protein: 2g (20%) Carbohydrate: 2g (5%) Fat: 5g (75%) Sodium: 5mg Potassium: 60mg Fiber: 1g

Garlic Herb Vinaigrette

This garlic herb vinaigrette provides a burst of flavor to your salads, with a delightful combination of aromatic herbs and zesty garlic.
Preparation Time: 5 minutes
Total Time: 5 minutes
Serving Size: 2 tablespoons
Ingredients:
2 tablespoons extra virgin olive oil
1 tablespoon apple cider vinegar
1 clove garlic, minced
1 teaspoon dried mixed herbs (such as basil, oregano, thyme)
Salt and pepper to taste
Directions:
1. In a small bowl, whisk together olive oil, apple cider vinegar, minced garlic, dried herbs, salt, and pepper.
2. Adjust seasonings to taste.
3. Transfer dressing into an airtight container and store in the fridge, use dressing within 5 days.
Nutritional Information (per serving): Calories: 90 Protein: 0g (0%) Carbohydrate: 1g (5%) Fat: 10g (80%) Sodium: 0mg Potassium: 10mg Fiber: 0g

Balsamic Dijon Dressing

This balsamic Dijon dressing offers a tangy and slightly sweet flavor, making it a versatile addition to your keto vegan salads.
Preparation Time: 5 minutes
Total Time: 5 minutes
Serving Size: 2 tablespoons
Ingredients:
2 tablespoons extra virgin olive oil
1 tablespoon balsamic vinegar
1 teaspoon Dijon mustard
1/2 teaspoon maple-flavored syrup substitute (for keto) or sweetener of choice
Salt and pepper to taste
Directions:
1. In a small bowl, whisk together olive oil, balsamic vinegar, Dijon mustard, sweetener, salt, and pepper until well combined.
2. Adjust seasonings to taste.
3. Transfer dressing into an airtight container and store in the fridge, use dressing within 5 days.

Nutritional Information (per serving): Calories: 70 Protein: 0g (0%) Carbohydrate: 1g (5%) Fat: 7g (80%) Sodium: 50mg Potassium: 10mg Fiber: 0g

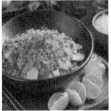

Ginger Sesame Dressing

This ginger sesame dressing offers a delightful blend of nutty and aromatic flavors, perfect for enhancing the taste of your keto vegan salads.
Preparation Time: 5 minutes
Total Time: 5 minutes
Serving Size: 2 tablespoons
Ingredients:
2 tablespoons toasted sesame oil
1 tablespoon rice vinegar (or apple cider vinegar for keto)
1 teaspoon grated fresh ginger
1 teaspoon tamari (or soy sauce substitute for keto)
1/2 teaspoon erythritol or preferred keto sweetener
Directions:
1. In a small bowl, whisk together toasted sesame oil, rice vinegar, grated ginger, tamari, and sweetener until well combined.
2. Adjust seasonings to taste.
3. Transfer dressing into an airtight container and store in the fridge, use dressing within 5 days.
Nutritional Information (per serving): Calories: 90 Protein: 0g (0%) Carbohydrate: 1g (5%) Fat: 10g (80%) Sodium: 150mg Potassium: 10mg Fiber: 0g

Creamy Garlic Almond Dressing

This creamy garlic almond dressing combines the rich, nutty flavor of almonds with the aromatic essence of garlic, providing a satisfying keto vegan option for your salads.
Preparation Time: 10 minutes
Total Time: 10 minutes
Serving Size: 2 tablespoons
Ingredients:
2 tablespoons almond butter
1 clove garlic, minced
2 tablespoons lemon juice
2 tablespoons water
Salt and pepper to taste
Directions:

1. In a small bowl, whisk together almond butter, minced garlic, lemon juice, water, salt, and pepper until well combined.
2. Adjust seasonings to taste. If needed, add more water for desired consistency.
3. Transfer dressing into an airtight container and store in the fridge, use dressing within 5 days.
Nutritional Information (per serving): Calories: 80 Protein: 2g (20%) Carbohydrate: 3g (7%) Fat: 7g (73%) Sodium: 5mg Potassium: 80mg Fiber: 2g

Herb Infused Olive Oil Dressing

This herb-infused olive oil dressing provides a burst of aromatic flavors, perfect for adding depth to your keto vegan salads.

Preparation Time: 5 minutes
Total Time: 5 minutes
Serving Size: 2 tablespoons

Ingredients:
2 tablespoons extra virgin olive oil
1 teaspoon dried mixed herbs (such as basil, rosemary, thyme)
1/2 teaspoon garlic powder
Salt and pepper to taste

Directions:
1. In a small bowl, whisk together extra virgin olive oil, dried herbs, garlic powder, salt, and pepper until well combined.
2. Adjust seasonings to taste.
3. Transfer dressing into an airtight container and store in the fridge, use dressing within 5 days.
Nutritional Information (per serving): Calories: 90 Protein: 0g (0%) Carbohydrate: 1g (5%) Fat: 10g (80%) Sodium: 0mg Potassium: 10mg Fiber: 0g

Creamy Lemon Chive Dressing

This creamy lemon chive dressing combines the zesty freshness of lemon with the mild, oniony flavor of chives, providing a delightful keto vegan option for your salads.

Preparation Time: 10 minutes
Total Time: 10 minutes
Serving Size: 2 tablespoons

Ingredients:
2 tablespoons vegan mayonnaise
1 tablespoon lemon juice
1 tablespoon chopped fresh chives
1/2 teaspoon Dijon mustard
Salt and pepper to taste

Directions:
1. In a small bowl, whisk together vegan mayonnaise, lemon juice, chopped chives, Dijon mustard, salt, and pepper until well combined.
2. Adjust seasonings to taste.
3. Transfer dressing into an airtight container and store in the fridge, use dressing within 5 days.

Nutritional Information (per serving): Calories: 80 Protein: 0g (0%) Carbohydrate: 1g (5%) Fat: 9g (80%) Sodium: 90mg Potassium: 10mg Fiber: 0g

Smoky Chipotle Dressing

This smoky chipotle dressing adds a spicy kick and a hint of smokiness to your salads, creating a bold and flavorful keto vegan option.

Preparation Time: 5 minutes

Total Time: 5 minutes

Serving Size: 2 tablespoons

Ingredients:

2 tablespoons olive oil

1 tablespoon lime juice

1 teaspoon chipotle pepper in adobo sauce, minced

1/2 teaspoon smoked paprika

Salt and pepper to taste

Directions:

1. In a small bowl, whisk together olive oil, lime juice, minced chipotle pepper, smoked paprika, salt, and pepper until well combined.

2. Taste dressing and make necessary adjustment as needed.

3. Transfer dressing into an airtight container and store in the fridge, use dressing within 5 days.

Nutritional Information (per serving): Calories: 70 Protein: 0g (0%) Carbohydrate: 1g (5%) Fat: 7g (80%) Sodium: 120mg\Potassium: 10mg Fiber: 0g

Creamy Cilantro Lime Dressing

This creamy cilantro lime dressing offers a burst of zesty and herby flavors, perfect for enhancing the taste of your keto vegan salads.

Preparation Time: 10 minutes

Total Time: 10 minutes

Serving Size: 2 tablespoons

Ingredients:

2 tablespoons vegan mayonnaise

1 tablespoon fresh lime juice

2 tablespoons chopped fresh cilantro

1 clove garlic, minced

Salt and pepper to taste

Directions:

1. In a small bowl, whisk together vegan mayonnaise, lime juice, chopped cilantro, minced garlic, salt, and pepper until well combined.

2. Taste dressing and make adjustment to suit your taste.

3. Transfer dressing into an airtight container and store in the fridge, use dressing within 5 days.

Nutritional Information (per serving): Calories: 80 Protein: 0g (0%) Carbohydrate: 1g (5%) Fat: 9g (80%) Sodium: 90mg Potassium: 10mg Fiber: 0g

Dill Ranch Dressing

This dill ranch dressing combines the creaminess of ranch with the fresh, herby flavor of dill, providing a delightful keto vegan option for your salads.
Preparation Time: 5 minutes
Total Time: 5 minutes
Serving Size: 2 tablespoons
Ingredients:
2 tablespoons vegan mayonnaise
1 tablespoon unsweetened almond milk
1 tablespoon chopped fresh dill
1/2 teaspoon garlic powder
Salt and pepper to taste
Directions:
1. In a small bowl, whisk together vegan mayonnaise, almond milk, chopped dill, garlic powder, salt, and pepper until well combined.
2. Taste dressing and make adjustment as needed.
3. Transfer dressing into an airtight container and store in the fridge, use dressing within 5 days.

Nutritional Information (per serving): Calories: 80 Protein: 0g (0%) Carbohydrate: 1g (5%) Fat: 9g (80%)\ Sodium: 90mg Potassium: 10mg Fiber: 0g

Turmeric Tahini Dressing

This turmeric tahini dressing offers a unique blend of earthy and nutty flavors, providing a vibrant keto vegan option for your salads.
Preparation Time: 5 minutes
Total Time: 5 minutes
Serving Size: 2 tablespoons
Ingredients:
2 tablespoons tahini
1 tablespoon lemon juice
1/2 teaspoon ground turmeric
1 tablespoon water
Salt to taste
Directions:
1. In a small bowl, whisk together tahini, lemon juice, ground turmeric, water, and salt until well combined.
2. Adjust water as needed for desired consistency.
3. Transfer dressing into an airtight container and store in the fridge, use dressing within 5 days.

Nutritional Information (per serving): Calories: 80 Protein: 2g (20%) Carbohydrate: 3g (7%) Fat: 7g (73%) Sodium: 5mg Potassium: 80mg Fiber: 1g

Spicy Peanut Dressing

This spicy peanut dressing combines the creaminess of peanut butter with a kick of heat, providing a bold and flavorful keto vegan option for your salads.

Preparation Time: 5 minutes
Total Time: 5 minutes
Serving Size: 2 tablespoons

Ingredients:
2 tablespoons peanut butter
1 tablespoon rice vinegar (or apple cider vinegar for keto)
1 teaspoon Sriracha sauce (adjust to taste)
1 tablespoon water
Salt to taste

Directions:
1. In a small bowl, whisk together peanut butter, vinegar, Sriracha sauce, water, and salt until well combined.
2. Adjust Sriracha and salt to taste.
3. Transfer dressing into an airtight container and store in the fridge, use dressing within 5 days.

Nutritional Information (per serving): Calories: 90 Protein: 3g (20%) Carbohydrate: 2g (5%) Fat: 8g (80%) Sodium: 100mg Potassium: 80mg Fiber: 1g

Creamy Cucumber Dill Dressing

This creamy cucumber dill dressing offers a refreshing and herby flavor, perfect for adding a cool touch to your keto vegan salads.

Preparation Time: 10 minutes
Total Time: 10 minutes
Serving Size: 2 tablespoons

Ingredients:
2 tablespoons vegan mayonnaise
2 tablespoons unsweetened almond milk
1/4 cup finely chopped cucumber
1 tablespoon chopped fresh dill
Salt and pepper to taste

Directions:
1. In a small bowl, whisk together vegan mayonnaise, almond milk, chopped cucumber, chopped dill, salt, and pepper until well combined.
2. Adjust seasonings to taste.
3. Transfer dressing into an airtight container and store in the fridge, use dressing within 5 days.

Nutritional Information (per serving): Calories: 60 Protein: 0g (0%) Carbohydrate: 2g (5%) Fat: 6g (80%) Sodium: 80mg Potassium: 10mg Fiber: 0g

Roasted Red Pepper and Walnut Dressing

This roasted red pepper and walnut dressing offers a rich and nutty flavor with a touch of smokiness, providing a unique keto vegan option for your salads.

Preparation Time: 15 minutes
Total Time: 15 minutes
Serving Size: 2 tablespoons
Ingredients:
1/4 cup roasted red peppers, drained
2 tablespoons walnuts
2 tablespoons extra virgin olive oil
1 tablespoon balsamic vinegar
Salt and pepper to taste
Directions:
1. In a blender or food processor, combine roasted red peppers, walnuts, olive oil, balsamic vinegar, salt, and pepper.
2. Blend until smooth and well combined.
3. Transfer dressing into an airtight container and store in the fridge, use dressing within 5 days.
Nutritional Information (per serving): Calories: 90 Protein: 1g (20%) Carbohydrate: 2g (5%) Fat: 9g (80%) Sodium: 85mg Potassium: 40mg Fiber: 1g

Printed in Great Britain
by Amazon

47353942R00066